Ageing Well

Quality of life
in old age

Growing Older
Series Editor: Alan Walker

The objective of this series is to showcase the major outputs from the ESRC Growing Older programme and to provide research insights which will result in improved policy and practice and enhanced and extended quality of life for older people.

It is well-known that people are living longer but until now very little attention has been given to the factors that determine the quality of life experienced by older people. This important new series will be vital reading for a broad audience of policy-makers, social gerontologists, nurses, social workers, sociologists and social geographers as well as advanced undergraduate and postgraduate students in these disciplines.

Series titles include:

Ann Bowling *Ageing Well*

Joanne Cook, Tony Maltby and Lorna Warren *Older Women's Lives*

Maria Evandrou and Karen Glaser *Family, Work and Quality of Life for Older People*

Mary Maynard, Haleh Afshar, Myfanwy Franks and Sharon Wray *Women in Later Life*

Sheila Peace, Caroline Holland and Leonie Kellaher *Environment and Identity in Later Life*

Thomas Scharf, Chris Phillipson and Allison E. Smith *Ageing in the City*

Christina Victor, Sasha Scambler and John Bond *The Social World of Older People*

Alan Walker (ed.) *Growing Older in Europe*

Alan Walker and Catherine Hagan Hennessy (eds) *Growing Older: Quality of Life in Old Age*

Alan Walker and Catherine Hagan Hennessy (eds) *Understanding Quality of Life in Old Age*

Ageing Well

Quality of life in old age

Ann Bowling

Open University Press

Open University Press
McGraw-Hill Education
McGraw-Hill House
Shoppenhangers Road
Maidenhead
Berkshire
England
SL6 2QL
email: enquiries@openup.co.uk
world wide web: www.openup.co.uk

and Two Penn Plaza, New York, NY 10121-2289, USA

First published 2005
Copyright © Ann Bowling 2005

A catalogue record of this book is available from the British Library

ISBN–10: 0335 21509 2 (pb) 0335 21510 6 (hb)
ISBN–13: 9780335215096 (pb) 9780335215102 (hb)

Library of Congress Cataloging-in-Publication Data
CIP data has been applied for

Typeset by RefineCatch Limited, Bungay, Suffolk
Printed in Poland EU by OZGraf. S.A.
www.polskabook.pl

Contents

Preface

I enjoy talking with very old men, for they have gone before us, as it were, on a road that we too may have to tread, and it seems to me that we should find out from them what it is like and whether it is rough and difficult or broad and easy.

Socrates, in Plato, The Republic, pp. 4–5, translated with an introduction by Desmond Lee, 1955, 2nd edn. 1987. © H.D.P. Lee. Reproduced with permission of Penguin Press.

There is international interest in how to improve the quality of human life while extending its quantity. But as Bond and Corner (2004) have pointed out, despite a long tradition in the sociology of ageing of eliciting and respecting lay views and perspectives, there are relatively few studies that have asked older people themselves about the quality of their lives. Hence the importance of the multi-method study presented here, which reports on older people's views of quality of life, and how it can be improved, as well as comparisons with the results of theoretically led measures of quality of life.

In this book I have presented data from a social survey of almost 1000 people aged 65 and over living at home in Britain: the *ESRC-MRC HSRC QoL Survey*. The research set out to discover what older people themselves thought about their lives and what is important to them, and especially how they rate their quality of life and how this can be improved. The findings enabled the 'drivers' of quality of life in older age to be identified, and key implications for policy-makers, and older people themselves, to be drawn up.

Chapter 1 presents an overview of the vast body of multi-disciplinary, theoretical and lay-based literature on the topic of quality of life. The methods of the study are presented in Chapter 2. I have organized the subsequent chapters containing the research findings around the quality of life themes mentioned by the older people themselves. In each chapter, following a more focused summary of the pertinent literature as an introduction, the quantitative data are presented as well as material from the open-ended survey questions and in-depth interviews. The latter clearly illustrate older people's perceptions of the things that gave their lives quality and the things that took quality away (material from the in-depth interviews is labelled as such, in order to distinguish it from the open-ended survey responses; the keys 'R' (respondent) and 'I' (interviewer) are used in the illustrations presented where applicable).

Acknowledgements

I am grateful to the Office for National Statistics (ONS) Omnibus Survey staff, and the ONS Qualitative Research Unit, in particular Maureen Kelly, Olwen Rowlands, Jack Eldridge and Kirsty Deacon for their much appreciated advice and help with designing the main survey questionnaire, for conducting focus groups with older people to inform the questionnaire design, for sampling and overseeing the Quality of Life Interview and processing the data. I would like to thank the ONS survey interviewers, Zahava Gabriel for her work on the in-depth interviews and their analysis, Priyha Solanki for assisting with the postal follow-up study, Joy Windsor and Matthew Bond for advice on statistical analysis, Anne Fleissig and Lee Marriott-Dowding for assistance with the open coding and the development of the coding frames, the transcribers of the audio-taped in-depth interviews, particularly Jessica Gregson, Deborah Elstein, Mark Freestone, Theo Lorenc and Ayse Ali, and the respondents themselves. Thanks also to Professor Robert Edelman, Mr Allan Brown, Mrs Marigold Brown and Dr Jackie Brown for suggesting illustrations. I am also grateful to Professor Stephen Sutton and Dr David Banister, the co-applicants for the ESRC Award which funded this research.

Those who carried out the original analysis and collection of the data hold no responsibility for the further analysis and interpretation of them. Material from the ONS Omnibus Survey, made available through ONS, has been used with the permission of the controller of The Stationery Office. The ONS Omnibus Survey dataset was deposited by ONS on the Data Archive at the University of Essex; the qualitative data was deposited by the research team on the Qualitative Data Archive, University of Essex. The author is also grateful to Baywood Publishing Company (*International Journal of Ageing and Mental Health*), Cambridge University Press (*Ageing and Society*), Carfax Publishing (*Ageing and Mental Health*), Springer Science and Business Media and Kluwer Academic Publishers (*Social Indicators Research*) for kind permission to reproduce some of the previously published material from the survey, including participants' quotations, and to Professor Alan Walker for permission to use material from a review of quality of life (copyrighted sources: Bowling, A., Banister, D. and Sutton, S. *et al.* (2002) A multidimensional model of QoL in older age, *Ageing and Mental Health*, 6: 355–71; Bowling, A., Gabriel, Z. and Dykes, J. *et al.* (2003) Let's ask them: a national survey of definitions of quality of life and its enhancement among people aged 65 and over, *International Journal of Aging and Human Development*, 56: 269–306; Bowling, A. and

Gabriel, Z. (2004) An integrational model of quality of life in older age: a comparison of analytic and lay models of quality of life, *Social Indicators Research*, 69: 1–36; Brown, J., Bowling, A. and Flyn, T. (2004) *Models of Quality of Life: A Taxonomy, Overview and Systematic Review of Quality of Life*, Sheffield: Department of Sociological Studies, European Forum on Population Ageing Research; Gabriel, Z. and Bowling, A. (2004b) Perspectives on quality of life in older age: older people talking, *Ageing and Society*, 24: 675–91).

The research was funded by the Economic and Social Research Council (ESRC) (award no. L480254003 (Quality of Life). The Quality of Life Questionnaire was also part-funded by grants, held collaboratively, by Professor Christina Victor and Professor John Bond (L480254042; Loneliness and Social Isolation, also part of the ESRC Growing Older Research Programme), and by Professor Shah Ebrahim (Medical Research Council Health Services Research Collaboration, Health and Disability).

Finally, the author gives special thanks to Professor Alan Walker, Director of the ESRC Growing Older (GO) Programme, and co-editor of this series on Growing Older, for his much motivating and greatly appreciated encouragement and support. Details of all the projects funded by the GO Programme can be found on the GO Programme website (http://www.shef.ac.uk/uni/projects/gop/index/htm).

Publications stemming from the research

Banister, D. and Bowling, A. (2004) Quality of life for the elderly – the transport dimension, *Transport Policy*, 11: 105–15.

Bowling, A. (in preparation) Quality of life – what older people say, in H. Mollenkopf and A. Walker (eds) *Quality of Life in Old Age: International and Multi-disciplinary Perspectives*. The Netherlands: Kluwer Academic Publishers.

Bowling, A. and Kennelly, C. (2003) *Adding Quality to Quantity: Older People's Views on Quality of Life and its Enhancement: Age Concern Reports*. London: Age Concern England.

Bowling, A. and Gabriel, Z. (2004) An integrational model of quality of life in older age: A comparison of analytic and lay models of quality of life, *Social Indicators Research*, 69: 1–36.

Bowling, A., Banister, D., Sutton, S., Evans, O. and Windsor, J. (2002) A multidimensional model of QoL in older age, *Ageing and Mental Health*, 6: 355–71.

Bowling, A., Gabriel, Z., Banister, D. and Sutton, S. (2002) Adding quality to quantity: older people's views on their quality of life and its enhancement, *ESRC Growing Older Programme: Research Findings*: 4.

Bowling, A., Gabriel, Z., Dykes, J., Marriott-Dowding, L., Fleissig, A., Evans, O., Banister, D. and Sutton, S. (2003) Let's ask them: a national survey of definitions of quality of life and its enhancement among people aged 65 and over, *International Journal of Aging and Human Development*, 56: 269–306.

Bowling, A., Seetai, S., Ebrahim, S., Gabriel, Z. and Solanki, P. (2005) Attributes of age-identity, *Ageing and Society*, 25: 479–500.

Brown, J., Bowling, A. and Flyn, T. (2004) *Models of Quality of Life: A taxonomy, Overview and Systematic Review of Quality of Life*. Sheffield: Department of Sociological Studies, European Forum on Population Ageing Research.

Gabriel, Z. and Bowling, A. (2004a) Perspectives on quality of life in older age: older people talking, *Ageing and Society* (Special Issue ESRC GO Programme commission), 24: 675–91.

Gabriel, Z. and Bowling, A. (2004b) Quality of life in older age from the perspectives of older people, in A. Walker and C. Hagen Hennessy (eds) *Growing Older: Quality of Life in Older Age*. Maidenhead: Open University Press.

List of abbreviations

ACE Age Concern England

Acorn A Classification of Residential Neighbourhoods

ADL activities of daily living

EuroQoL European Quality of Life (questionnaire)

IADL instrumental activities of daily living

GHQ-12 General Health Questionnaire, 12-item version

GO Growing Older Programme

GSS General Social Survey

HRQoL health-related quality of life

LSI long-standing illness (including disability, infirmity)

LLSI Limitations due to LSI

ONS Office for National Statistics

QoL quality of life

SEIQoL Schedule for the Evaluation of Individual Quality of Life

SES socioeconomic status

SIR social indicators research

SOC selective optimization with compensation

SF-36 Short-Form 36 Health Survey

WHO World Health Organization

WHOQoL World Health Organization Quality of Life (group and questionnaire)

1

Models of quality of life in older age

'When I use a word,' Humpty Dumpty said in rather a scornful tone, 'it means just what I choose it to mean – neither more nor less.' 'The question is,' said Alice, 'whether you can make words mean so many different things.'

Lewis Carroll, *Through the Looking Glass* (1872: 274)

Background

The increasing number of people living longer has led to international interest in the enhancement of quality of life (QoL) and health-related quality of life (HRQoL) in older age. This interest is unsurprising as demographic changes have been remarkable. In Britain, for example, in 1951, 16% of the population was aged 60 or over; 50 years on this had risen to 21% (Office for National Statistics 2003). By 2050 around one person in five (12 million) will be aged over 70, and a further 8 million will be in their 60s. Predictions are that average life expectancy, between 2001 and 2026, will rise from 75.6 years to 79 years for men, and from 80.4 years to 83.3 years for women (Office for National Statistics 2004). Population projections predict that the number of people on retirement pensions will exceed the number of children for the first time in 2007 (Office for National Statistics 2003). Older people will thus be a far more important group politically (number of votes) in their own right, in terms of spending power, and as consumers of services.

Interest in QoL and ageing, and maintaining independence among older people, has been fuelled by policy concerns to reduce public expenditure on pensions, health and social welfare provisions, and by higher expectations in society of achieving and maintaining 'a good life'. The hypothesized future compression of morbidity and disability into a shorter period of life, with greater healthy or disability-free life expectancy is leading to more positive perspectives of healthy ageing as normal, although the evidence in support of this is stronger in the USA than in Britain, and there is still debate over measurement and interpretation (Péron 1992; Manton *et al.* 1993, 1995; Grundy 1997; Dunnell and Dix 2000; Kelly and Baker 2000). However, public policy is increasingly likely to be concerned with enabling older people to maintain their mobility, independence, their active contribution to society, and to respond effectively to the challenges of older age. The interest in QoL has not been confined to issues of ageing. There has been an enormous increase in publications on well-being and QoL over the last few decades (Fernàndez-Ballesteros 1998a, 2003). Attempts are also being made to develop item banks of calibrated QoL scales and more sensitive, standardized assessments of QoL (Ware and Bayliss 2003).

The move away from negative models of ageing

This all reflects a shift of emphasis away from a negative paradigm of old age, and towards a positive view of old age as a natural component of the life span (O'Boyle 1997) – as a period of life in which one is free from many structured social roles, able to explore areas of personal fulfilment and social activity, and in good health (Roizen 1999; Willcox *et al.* 2001; World Health Organization 2002; Huber and Skidmore 2003; Roizen and Stephenson 2003). Of course, in reality, limited resources, opportunity and ill-health can be restrictive, but there is still an overall focus on demolishing stereotypes of older age.

With the earlier negative, 'pathology' model, a main focus of social and clinical research, particularly in Europe, encompassed issues of dependency, poverty, service use and care needs, and declining physical and mental health (Bowling 1993). This was at the expense of enablement, rehabilitation, prevention and cure (Roos and Havens 1991). The positivist perspective of functionalism also influenced the development of narrow, proxy QoL scales in the social and health care field. This reinforced a negative concentration on physical and psychological functioning (i.e. inability to do things; depression and anxiety) at the expense of the positive (i.e. ability, happiness). Research based on this model has inevitably underestimated the QoL of older people.

Heterogeneity among older people

There is great heterogeneity among older people, which population figures and projections camouflage. There is also increasing awareness that physical and mental decline is not an inevitable part of the third or fourth ages. Indeed, there is no consensus about what constitutes 'old'. Any categorization by age obscures the diversity of older people, physiologically, psychologically and socially. Although it is important not to get the association between disability and advanced old age out of perspective, most older people in their 60s and 70s are independent, engage in everyday activities without major restrictions, and most report that they are happy and satisfied with their lives (Bowling *et al.* 1991, 1999; Walker and Maltby 1997). While for some, older age will be a time of increasing dependency and loss of control, for others it will be a period of personal fulfilment. While sociodemographic characteristics can be important sources of differentiation among older people, and can influence the experience of ageing (Grundy and Bowling 1997), even philosophers long ago recognized that older age also contains many opportunities for positive change and productive functioning, and should not be confused with illness (Cicero 44 BC, reprinted 1979).

Social theories of ageing

There are three major social theories of ageing which have been of relevance to research on QoL in older age: disengagement theory, activity theory and continuity theory (see Box 1.1), but each of these has been subject to criticism, and they are now seen as dated products of their era (Putnam 2002). The study of ageing was given impetus by post-war health and social policy concerns regarding demographic changes, and by a political economy which regarded an ageing population as problematic. This stemmed from functionalist theory which argued that the well-being of society required the maintenance of

---

Box 1.1 Social theories of ageing

Disengagement theory: gradual withdrawal from social interactions and activities is an inevitable accompaniment of older age; this protects the individual against the trauma of dying and minimizes disruption to society when death takes place (Cumming and Henry 1961).

Activity, or role, theory: maintenance of social roles and activities that are meaningful to people enhance feelings of well-being in older age (Havighurst and Albrecht 1953; Lemon *et al.* 1972).

Continuity theory: individuals make adaptations to enable them to feel the continuity between the past and present, which preserves their psychological well-being (Atchley 1989, 1999).

---

functions – education, family, religion, government. Of course, functionalism reflected culturally dominant perspectives of the time, but it produced the *then* powerful theories of disengagement, activity and continuity.

Disengagement theory was weak in so far as it assumed that disengagement was a desirable state, and it ignored the role of the political economy in forcing withdrawal from society. It gradually became outdated, given increasing evidence of the socially active lives being pursued by most older people, with benefits to their well-being and morale (Maddox 1963), although social activity in older age is associated with socioeconomic group, with those higher up the social scale enjoying the highest levels of social participation (Marmot *et al.* 2003). The counterpoint to disengagement theory was activity theory, which held that 'successful' or 'positive' ageing could be achieved by maintaining roles and relationships, not by withdrawing from them. Activity theory was too simplistic, however, and ignored issues of social inequality, and associations between deteriorating health and functioning, losses to social networks (e.g. through bereavement) and reduced social activity. Continuity theory proposed a need for internal (self-concept) and external (social roles, activities, relationships and so on) consistency in people's lives, and a process of continuous development and adaptation throughout life in response to life events and changes. But this was also over-simplistic and ignored issues of power and inequality in society.

Social system theories of ageing

More realistic are some of the theories of ageing within the social system, such as social exchange theory, modernization theory and age stratification theory (see Box 1.2), as they recognize the economic and political forces that have led to the inequality and ageism experienced by older people, and which can detract from their QoL. But social system theories, and the empirical studies deriving from them, have been criticized for their ahistoricism – the implicit assumption of a linear progression from primitive to modern society – and the failure to recognize the diversity of social structures in the developed world (Grundy and Bowling 1997).

Other theories focus on the political economy of ageing (focusing on political, economic and social structures) including feminist perspectives and power differentials in society (e.g. based on age). However, each of these theories neglects key areas of concern to individuals and key themes within ageing (Putnam 2002). Neglected issues of dependency, disability and social handicaps were partly redressed by the theory of structured dependency.

Box 1.2 Social system theories of ageing

Social exchange theory: the cost-benefit ratio between the individual and society falls out of balance in older age, thus the costs of interacting with older people outweigh the benefits (Dowd 1975).

Modernization theory: with the emergence of new technology, which undermined the status of older people through the emphasis on education, rather than older adults passing on knowledge and skills, older adults lost their place of prestige and power within the social system (Burgess 1960).

Age stratification theory: there is an age structure to roles, and normative age criteria for certain activities, thus with age a cohort moves to a different set of roles as a younger generation takes its place (Riley *et al.* 1972).

For example, Walker (1981) argued the case for a 'political economy of old age' in order to better understand the situation of older people, and in particular the 'social creation of dependency' – the development of dependency due to restricted access to societal resources, including income. Attention has also been focused on models of environmental fit and the creation of dependency (the balance between environmental demands and individual capabilities, such as when a person can no longer climb stairs and thus relocates living space all on one floor or seeks help – Lawton and Nahemow 1973). These issues are of great importance, and can affect the QoL of older people.

The low status of older people in advanced industrial societies has been attributed to modern, post-industrial capitalism. The state is held responsible for the creation of structured dependency, in which statutory exit from the labour market at retirement age leads to marginalization from social and economic life, and forced dependence on low pension provisions (Walker 1981). Recent concerns about labour shortages internationally, however, have led to some rethinking of this policy. There is no reason for deciding that the whole population suddenly loses the capacity for productive work at a fixed age, and retirement policies are likely to reinforce the marginalization of those over a certain age. Not all the problems of older people can be blamed on late twentieth-century retirement policies however, with retirement policies documented in the sixth century, and age-related retirement policies in the USA and several European countries affecting around a third of the male urban workforce by the late nineteenth century (see Grundy and Bowling 1997). While there are several relatively crude presentations and critiques of the political economy of ageing thesis, Walker (in press) has reviewed these and critically discussed the continuing relevance of the approach.

However, while social structures may threaten well-being, individual experiences are derived from interrelated levels of social structure, such as social stratification (including age stratification), social institutions and interpersonal relationships (Pearlin 1989), together with individual personality and psychological influences (see p. 8). This suggests that models of ageing need to be broad and cross disciplines, rather than being rooted inflexibly within any single model.

Positive approaches to ageing

A retirement lifestyle has emerged with a focus on health and liberation, as opposed to illness and disability (Blaikie 1999), and there has been a gradually increasing emphasis on the achievement of positive, healthy, well, active or 'successful ageing' (Butt and Beiser 1987; Berkman et al. 1992; Fisher 1992, 1995; Fisher et al. 1992; Bearon 1996; Fisher and Specht 1999; Andrews et al. 2002; World Health Organization 2002; Baltes and Smith 2003; Phelan et al. 2004). The influence of earlier functionalist perspectives on achieving this lingers in definitions which emphasize that successful ageing is achieved through adaptation and adjustment to socially acceptable role changes.

There are numerous definitions of successful ageing. These include: having the physiological and psychological abilities of younger people, and engaging with life (Rowe and Kahn 1987, 1998, 1997); reaching one's potential and achieving physical, psychological and social well-being (Gibson 1995); the ability to adapt one's values to meet the challenges of later life (Clark and Andersson 1967); maintaining a realistic sense of self (Brandstadter and Greve 1994); employing various compensatory and accommodative strategies in the face of depleting reserves; cognitive efficiency; psychological resources built up over a lifetime; self-mastery; control; maintenance of productivity; achievement (Baltes and Baltes 1990a, 1990b; Baltes et al. 1996); and, simply, a sense of *being*, coupled with optimum functioning (von Faber et al. 2001). There is some supportive evidence that these strategies are associated with higher levels of life satisfaction and QoL (Freund and Baltes 1998). The achievement and maintenance of life satisfaction has also been identified, together with physical health status, as essential for 'successful ageing' (Vaillant 1990, 2002). However, mirroring research on QoL, there is evidence that older people hold broader views of 'successful ageing' than these (Brandstadter and Greve 1994; Strawbridge *et al.* 1996; Tate *et al.* 2003). Older people themselves include social activities, interests and goals in their definitions. There is also little empirical support for Tornstam's (1997) view that people develop a more transcendent perspective of life with older age. The concept of 'successful ageing' has been subject to much criticism because it is embedded in North American value systems of success or failure (Torres 1999, 2003), rather than on individuals' values.

There is more emphasis in current models of ageing on life-span influences. These examine socioeconomic status over time, and influences on current health and psychosocial circumstances. Life-span models also focus on behaviour, and the positive benefits of physical exercise, lifestyle factors, cognitively stimulating activities, and maintaining an optimistic outlook for future health and well-being (Hartman-Stein and Potkanowicz 2003). In theory, these all have implications for achieving quality of later life.

Models of QoL in older age

Given its popularity as an endpoint in the evaluation of public policy (e.g. outcomes of health and social care), a multi-faceted perspective of QoL is required which reflects the views of the population concerned. QoL theoretically encompasses the individual's physical health, psychosocial well-being and functioning, independence, control over life, material circumstances and the external environment. It is a concept which is dependent on the perceptions of individuals, and is likely to be mediated by cognitive factors (WHOQOL Group 1993; Skevington 1999; Skevington *et al.* 1999; Bowling 2001).

QoL thus reflects both macro, societal, and micro, individual, influences, and it is a collection of objective and subjective dimensions which interact together (Lawton 1991), with theoretical distinctions between the liveability of the environment (social capital), the individual (personal capacities and psychological capital), the external utility of life and inner appreciation of life (Veenhoven 2000). For example, Lawton (1982, 1983a, 1983b) argued that well-being in older people may be represented by behavioural and social competence (e.g. measured by indicators of health, cognition, time use and social behaviour); perceived quality of life (measured by the individual's subjective evaluation of each domain of life); psychological well-being (measured by indicators of mental health, cognitive judgements of life satisfaction, positive-negative emotions); and the external, objective (physical) environment (housing and economic indicators). He thus developed a quadripartite concept of the 'good life' for older people (Lawton 1983a), which he later changed to 'quality of life' as the preferred overall term, accounting for all of life. The model is still popular and has been recently tested in Europe and reported to successfully discriminate between older Swedish and Polish populations (Jaracz *et al.* 2004).

Most disciplines have based their concepts and measures on experts' opinions, rather than those of lay people (Rogerson *et al.*, 1989a, 1989b; Bowling 2001). This has the consequence that there is little empirical data on the extent to which the items included in most measurement scales have any relevance to people and their everyday lives. In addition, a pragmatic approach prevails in the literature, and clarification of the concept of QoL is typically bypassed, and justified with reference to its abstract nature, and the selection of measurement scales often appears ad hoc (Carver *et al.* 1999). Moreover, models of quality of life are not consistent. Some have incorporated a needs-based satisfaction model, based on Maslow's (1954, 1968) hierarchy of human needs for maintenance and existence (physiological, safety and security, social and belonging, ego, status and self-esteem, and self-actualization). Scales used to measure the QoL of people with mental health problems, for example, are based on a satisfaction of human needs model, coupled with assessments of global well-being (Bowling 2001). Higgs *et al.* (2003) also based their model of QoL in older age on self-actualization and self-esteem. In contrast, traditional US social science models of quality of life have been based primarily on the overlapping, positive, concepts of 'the good life', 'life satisfaction', 'social well-being', 'morale', 'the social temperature' or 'happiness' (Andrews and Withey 1976a, 1976b; Andrews 1986). This reflects the influence of early Greek and nineteenth-century utilitarian philosophy, with a focus on well-being, happiness, pleasure and satisfaction.

Social gerontologists, particularly in the USA, have continued to emphasize this positive, subjective perspective by highlighting the importance of psychological resources in older age, including:

◆ adaptability;

◆ autonomy;

◆ activity;

◆ cognitive competence;

◆ control over life;

◆ life satisfaction;

- morale;

- optimization and compensatory strategies;

- personal growth;

- retention of independence;

- self-efficacy;

- social role functioning;

- well-being.

These areas have all been suggested as key constituents of QoL (Larson 1978; Andrews 1986; Baltes and Baltes 1990b; Day 1991; Fisher 1995; Lawton 1996; Fry 2000). With optimization and compensatory strategies (Baltes and Baltes 1990b), ageing is seen through a life-course perspective, as an ongoing process involving and interplay between selection (as restrictions are imposed on activities, people 'select' areas of highest priority), optimization (people maintain behaviours that augment their physical and mental reserves, in order to maximize their chosen way of life) and compensation (people compensate by using psychological and technological strategies). This dynamic theory of developmental change and resilience across the life span holds that by using these strategies a person can maximize the positive and minimize the negative outcomes of older age (Freund and Baltes 1998; Freund and Riediger 2003).

The taxonomy of models of QoL, compiled previously by this author (see Brown *et al.* 2004), included models based on a wide range of concepts (see Box 1.3). An overview of these main models of QoL will be presented in the next section.

Box 1.3 Taxonomy of models of QoL

- Objective indicators
- Subjective indicators
- Satisfaction of human needs
- Psychological characteristics and resources
- Health and functioning
- Social health
- Social cohesion and social capital
- Environmental context
- Idiographic approaches

Overview of models of quality of life

Objective indicators

The objective approach is essentially a needs-based approach, which assumes that there are basic needs in society, and that satisfying these needs determines people's well-being (Delhey *et al.* 2002). This perspective, with a focus on living conditions and material resources, is prevalent in Scandinavian countries (Erikson 1993; Noll and Zapf 1994; Johansson 2002; Noll 2002a; Veenhoven 2002), although many other countries also monitor key indicators of living circumstances (e.g. Department for Environment, Food and Rural Affairs 2002).

It has been argued that objective indicators are essential in order to make uniform assessments of people's circumstances, and of met and unmet needs, which are undistorted by individuals' perceptions (Meeberg 1993). Critical social gerontology in Europe holds that QoL is influenced as much by objective social and economic circumstances as by the characteristics of the individual. While some investigators defined *objective*, or non-experiential, indicators in terms of measurable cost of living and other economic indictors ('facts'), including income, work and unemployment figures, others have broadened this to include objective data which encompass all circumstances of life and living conditions. These include type of housing tenure/home ownership, ownership of consumer durables, overcrowding, leisure activities, social participation, health, environment and pollution, crime levels, education, social class, age, gender and so on (Flax 1972; Campbell *et al.* 1976; Wingo and Evans 1978; Rogerson *et al.* 1989a, 1989b; Sherman and Schiffman 1991; Boelhouwer 2002; Muntaner and Lynch 2002).

Veenhoven (1999), on the basis of national comparisons from the World Database of Happiness, which indicated that the more individualized the nation, the more citizens enjoyed their lives, added 'individualization of society' to the list, including indicators of individualistic values; people's capability to choose (measured by indicators of education and information); opportunities for freedom of political choice (political and civil rights, including democratic rights); freedom of economic choice (security of finances, freedom to produce and consume what one wants, freedom to keep what one earns and freedom of exchange); and freedom of personal choices (e.g. choice in divorce, abortion and so on).

Associations with objective indicators

The most consistent associations between objective variables and indicators of well-being across Europe and the USA are with health and functional status, particularly among older people (although these are often measured subjectively using self-rating scales and cannot be classified strictly as objective), and with level of income (Kushman and Lane 1980; Usui *et al.* 1985; Markides and Martin 1979; Waters *et al.* 1998). Blanchflower and Oswald (2001), in their time series analyses of US and British subjective data, reported that not only was reported happiness associated with higher income and being employed, but it was also greater for women, married people and the more highly educated. Gender may also indirectly influence QoL as older women are more likely than men to be widowed and to live alone, and to have poorer physical functioning, even when controlling for socioeconomic status (Haug and Folmar 1986). Studies of ageing have found strong associations between indicators of socioeconomic inequality, perceived well-being and morale among older people (e.g. Breeze *et al.* 2001). However, the data on income and well-being is not straightforward, and it has been found that huge increases in wealth are required to influence feelings of happiness (Gardner and Oswald 2001) (see section on relative deprivation, below). It has also been reported elsewhere that the more educated are also the least satisfied with their QoL, and have reduced feelings of well-being, perhaps because they have higher expectations of the rewards of education which are not always met (supporting relative deprivation theory that as education increases people's relative expectations and potential for dissatisfaction also increases) (Clark and Oswald 1996; Olson 1996; Oswald and Frank 1997; Bowling and Windsor 2001; Frey and Stutzer 2001). Less attention has been paid to neighbourhood characteristics and well-being, although there is some evidence that rural living and social integration affects satisfaction and well-being (Lawton 1980; Wenger 1984a, 1984b).

Relative deprivation

Research has often cast doubt on the power of objective variables alone in predicting QoL ratings, especially in view of the paradox of well-being – the presence of subjective well-being in the face of objective difficulties which would be expected to predict unhappiness (Mroczek and Kolarz 1998). Diener and Biswas-Myers (2002) reported data documenting that people are happier if they live in wealthy rather than poor nations. Veenhoven (1991, 1993, 1994), Oswald and Frank (1997), Blanchflower and Oswald (2001) and Ehrhardt *et al.* (2000) have all presented data showing that greater happiness is associated with better living conditions, affluence and income. But, while income plays an important role in determining life expectancy, happiness and well-being (Darnton-Hill 1995), and there is evidence that one's outlook is associated with the place occupied in the status hierarchy (Marmot 2004), most studies have reported high levels of well-being and happiness regardless of economic circumstances (Easterlin 1974, 1995; Headey and Wearing 1992; and see James 1997, 2003). In addition, no differences were found in QoL between deprived and more affluent communities in the USA (Smith 2000). Relative deprivation theory is supported by this research. It has also been shown that wealth may even adversely affect happiness (Kasser 2002). Easterlin (1974, 1995) argued that people obtain utility (i.e. satisfaction) by comparing themselves with others close to them; as affluence and education increases, people's relative expectations and potential for dissatisfaction increases (see p. 11; Clark and Oswald 1996; Olsen 1996; Oswald and Frank 1997).

While the concept of relative deprivation is contentious (Veenhoven 1991; Headey and Wearing 1992), only small to moderate correlations, at best, between objective indicators, including income and sociodemographic characteristics, and satisfaction with life, happiness, well-being or QoL ratings have been reported (Campbell *et al.* 1976; Lehman 1983; Inglehart and Rabier 1986; Michalos and Zumbo 2000; Bowling and Windsor 2001).

One explanation for the relatively low predictive power of objective variables alone is their very omission of a subjective element which taps how these areas affect a person's life. It has also been argued that QoL is additive, reflecting the sum of one's experience, adjustment and satisfaction in several domains of life (Inglehart and Rabier 1986). Or possibly they are less relevant, and therefore have less explanatory power, in societies which have achieved a certain level of affluence, and subjective perceptions, social expectations and comparisons (see above and p. 21) become more influential. Heylighten and Bernheim (2000) have defined the dimensions that make up well-being and QoL, including happiness, as the sum of mainly relative subjective factors but with a small contribution from objective factors. In addition, the collection and interpretation of objective 'facts' is also subject to a series of subjective biases, errors, inaccuracies, and political and perceptual influences. Defenders of the objective approach argue that the data is needed to inform social policy, undistorted by and independent of, public opinion surveys which can reflect random errors and biases (Johansson 2002). Burholt (2001) has summarized some of this literature, and emphasizes the need for a multi-dimensional approach. Saris (1996) proposed a compromise perspective and argued that QoL is the sum of absolute, objective factors (reflecting living situations) and relative, subjective factors (reflecting a person's aspirations). This helps to explain why objective factors, while correlating significantly with subjective well-being (Heylighten and Bernheim 2000), are weak overall predictors of life satisfaction or overall QoL assessments in multi-variate models (Bowling and Windsor 2001).

In sum, while relative deprivation theory appears powerful, the underlying importance of income should not be underestimated (Darnton-Hill 1995). Adequate income has implications for health, standard of housing, education, nutrition, clothing, transport, opportunities for leisure and social participation. In a national population survey of the most important areas of life, financial and living circumstances were self-nominated by about six in ten of all adult respondents, although its perceived importance decreased with age, with 48% of those aged 65<75 and 35% of those aged 75+ self-nominating it (Bowling 1995a, 1995b, 1996; Bowling and Windsor 2001). And, particularly in relation to older people, the influence of level of income reflects both past income, present income and accumulated income over the life-course. But while life-course influences can be strong, and influence the present, actual current circumstances themselves can have a stronger impact on people's well-being and perceptions (Blane *et al.* 2002).

Subjective indicators

In contrast to objective indicators, subjective indicators are those which involve some evaluation (e.g. expression of (dis-)satisfaction, values and perceptions) of one's circumstances in life. It is unlikely that human happiness and satisfaction can be understood fully without asking people about their feelings. Subjective, or experiential, social indicators are based on the model of subjective well-being as defined by people's 'hedonic feelings or cognitive satisfactions' (Diener and Suh 1997). People are routinely engaged in evaluating themselves in relation to the life domains they consider to be of relevance, and important, to themselves. Subjective indicators institutionalize, or formalize, these natural tendencies. Subjective indicators include measures of life satisfaction and psychological well-being, morale, individual fulfilment and happiness, balance of affect and self-worth (esteem) (Gurin *et al.* 1960; Bradburn and Caplowitz 1965; Bradburn 1969; Andrews 1973; Andrews and Withey 1976a, 1976b; Campbell *et al.* 1976; Bigelow *et al.* 1982; Lawton 1983a, 1983b; Rosenwaike 1985; Ryff 1989a, 1989b; Day 1991; Roos and Havens 1991; Suzman *et al.* 1992; Garfein and Herzog 1995; Clarke *et al.* 2000).

Making an overall judgement about the quality of one's life implies a cognitive, intellectual activity and requires the assessment of past experiences and estimation of future experiences: 'Both require a marshalling of facts into a convenient number of cognitive categories. It also demands an evaluation of priorities and relative values' (Veenhoven 1991). Quality of life assessment is also bipolar, consisting of the independent dimensions of positive and also negative affect. The difficulty for research lies in capturing the relevant and important areas to most people. While social desirability and other biases inevitably threaten subjective measures (Hughes 1990; Schwartz and Strack 1999; Johansson 2002; Veenhoven 2002), researchers have risen to the challenge with exhaustive, now classic investigations of the validity of their measures (Andrews and Crandall 1976). It is now commonly accepted that objective living conditions and subjective evaluations of personal life circumstances are just two sides of the same coin (Delhey *et al.* 2002), and both now tend to be included as indicators of life quality, happiness and well-being (Argyle 1996; Hudler and Richter 2002). Despite potential biases, subjective indicators are still needed in the setting of policy goals, based on what people need and want, and evaluations of success require public support (Veenhoven 2002). Objective indicators alone do not provide sufficient information.

Social indicators research

The social indicators research (SIR) movement emerged in the 1960s in the USA, and later in parts of Europe as a reaction to the traditional reliance on economic indicators to tap society's well-being, and the then dominant post-war, societal goal of increasing materialism. It developed momentum in response to the awareness of poverty in affluent societies (Johansson 2002) and gradually diversified and focused on the collection of wider objective indicators for social monitoring and tapping QoL. Noll (2002b) dated the movement from the mid-1960s and the efforts made by the American space agency (NASA) to assess the impact of the American space programme on US society. He credited the director of the project with the initial definition and use of the concept 'social indicator' as 'statistics, statistical series, and all other forms of evidence that enable us to assess where we stand and are going with respect to our values and goals' (Bauer 1966). The United Nations (1994) extended this activity to the use of the indicators in identification of problems and policy priority setting.

Gradually, the balance of the focus in the USA was tipped towards subjective, experiential indicators as outcome indicators (e.g. Andrews and Withey 1976a; Campbell *et al.* 1976). Andrews and Withey argued that the perception and evaluation of life by people is important when monitoring QoL, for example their judgements on crime levels, as well as their evaluations of more private aspects of their lives (see section on well-being, p. 16). In contrast, as previously pointed out, in Europe the focus of gerontology was still less theoretically based, and more focused on older people's objective social and economic circumstances, and subjective assessments limited to needs for health and social care (Hughes 1990).

However, the increasingly diverse SIR movement generally failed to influence politics and planning, and was also discontinued in many countries (e.g. the Organization for Economic Cooperation and Development – OECD – programmes terminated in the 1980s). Governments instead started to develop their own information systems and standardized social surveys to monitor living conditions. There has been increasing interest in the identification of national QoL indexes with policy relevance (Hagerty et al. 2001), and an explosion of surveys, which have collected both objective and subjective data on QoL nationally and internationally (Blanchflower and Oswald 2001; Audit Commission 2002; Delhey et al. 2002; Department for Environment, Food and Rural Affairs 2002; Hudler and Richter 2002; Noll 2002b; Pfizer 2002; Mercer Human Resource Consulting 2003; Moriarty et al. 2003; Economist Intelligence Unit 2004; Hagerty et al. 2004). Despite this more integrative approach, a tension between subjective and objective approaches remains in European countries (Walker 2005), with objective measures being used more frequently.

Perceptual needs satisfaction models

A needs-based satisfaction model of QoL has been derived from Maslow's (1954, 1968) hierarchy of shared human needs which are judged to be necessary for maintenance and existence:

- physiological;
- safety and security;
- social and belonging;
- ego;
- status and self-esteem;
- self-actualization.

Maslow (1968) proposed that once basic needs are satisfied, human beings pursue higher needs such as self-actualization, happiness and esteem. Hörnquist (1982) argued that human needs are the foundations for QoL, and hence QoL can be defined in terms of human needs and the satisfactory fulfilment of those needs (e.g. physical, psychological, social, activity, marital and structural). Basic needs satisfaction is, of course, of importance to vulnerable groups in society. Satisfaction of needs for personal care, food and safety were among older people's top five priorities for inclusion in the outcome measurement of social care, the others being social participation, involvement in, and control over, daily life (Netten *et al.* 2002). As pointed out earlier (p. 8) most scales used to measure the QoL of people with mental health problems are based on perceptions of satisfaction with levels of met needs (Lehman 1988; Bigelow *et al.* 1991; Bowling 2004a); the former include a person's subjective evaluations of their (satisfaction with) objective circumstances, including access to information and advice, money, tangible goods and services, as well as subjective circumstances such as love and status (Rettig and Leichtentritt 1999). Of course, 'satisfaction' in this context can again be influenced by social comparisons and expectations (Sirgy 1998) (see p. 21). Others have argued that a sense of purpose, self-esteem and self-worth are also crucial for good QoL, including QoL in people with dementia (Sarvimäki 1999). Hyde *et al.* (2003) based their assessment of QoL on a needs satisfaction model, focusing on the higher needs of control, autonomy, pleasure and self-realization, and reported that their measure correlated highly with life satisfaction (and see Higgs *et al.* 2003).

Psychological and personality models

Subjective well-being, life satisfaction and happiness

Traditional social science models of QoL in North America have been based primarily on the overlapping concepts of 'the good life', 'life satisfaction', 'social well-being', 'morale' 'the social temperature' and 'happiness' (Andrews and Withey 1976a; Andrews 1986). Morale and well-being have been the most frequently explored proxy variables of QoL, generally defined and measured in terms of life satisfaction, morale and self-esteem, sometimes supplemented with narrower scales of psychological morbidity (Wenger 1992; Bowling 2004a).

However, while terms overlap, QoL is conceptually distinct from well-being, morale, life satisfaction and so on (Spiro and Bossé 2000). Of concern, both theoretically and methodologically, is the interchangeable use, without justification, of all these distinct concepts. These concepts are commonly measured using one of a small number of overlapping scales (Andrews and Withey 1976a; Antonovsky 1987; Bradburn 1969; Campbell *et al.* 1976; Cantril 1967;

Dupuy 1984, 1978; Kutner *et al.* 1956; Lawton 1972, 1975; Michalos 1991; Neugarten *et al.* 1961; Wood *et al.* 1969). The selection of measures of life satisfaction, morale and affect is often made without theoretical justification or attempts to fit a pre-defined model, despite the fact that a scale measuring life satisfaction cannot adequately measure the other related but distinct concepts. Awareness of the distinctions between all these concepts is necessary when interpreting data. For example, older people often report lower levels of happiness than younger people, but report higher levels of life satisfaction and positive affect with older age (Campbell *et al.* 1976; Campbell 1981; Mroczek and Kolarz 1998) – although this is lower among very elderly people (Bowling *et al.* 1991). Of course, 'old age' can span over 30 years of a lifetime, and older people are as heterogeneous in their perceived well-being as younger people, if not more (Stewart *et al.* 1996).

Subjective well-being   In the developed world, QoL has been equated with perceived well-being, namely the extent to which pleasure and happiness, and ultimately satisfaction with life, have been obtained (Andrews 1974). This reflects the influence of early Greek and nineteenth-century utilitarian philosophy, focusing on hedonistic aspects of life – the maximization of well-being, happiness, pleasure and satisfaction – and Bentham's ([1834] 1983) utilitarian philosophy, which regarded well-being as the difference in value between the sum of all pleasures and the sum of all pains, and argued that society should aim for the greatest good of the greatest number.

Subjective, or emotional, well-being consists of people's own evaluations of their lives (Diener and Lucas 2000), either cognitive (e.g. specific or overall life satisfaction) or affective (e.g. feelings of joy) (Andrews and Withey 1976a). The concept can be divided into state (current well-being) and trait (well-being as feature of character). Warr (1999) postulated that self-reported well-being measures reflect at least four factors: circumstances, aspirations, comparisons with others and a person's baseline happiness or disposition. In contrast to positive psychologists who argue that optimism can be learned in order to enhance one's well-being, it has been reported from genetic studies of twins that there is likely to be a large dispositional effect on perceived well-being (Lykken and Tellegen 1996).

Well-being is usually defined, then, in terms of satisfaction with overall and current life, and happiness. 'Overall subjective well-being' measures consist of individuals' assessments of their lifetime, or expected stock value or flow, of future utilities (Blanchflower and Oswald 2001). 'Current well-being' measures focus on current circumstances (Sarvimäki and Stonbock-Hult 2000). Investigators of well-being often use multi-dimensional measures, but rarely clarify the different concepts used to denote well-being (Wenger 1989; Wenger and Shahtahmasebi 1990). The concept has also been used as an indicator of HRQoL, although it has been shown to be conceptually distinct (Ranzijn and Luszcz 2000; Spiro and Bossé 2000).

Life satisfaction   Life satisfaction, then, is commonly taken to denote well-being, and was an early social indicator of QoL (Andrews and Withey 1976a; Campbell *et al.* 1976). It is a cognitive judgement, or assessment, of one's life overall (made up of assessments of its component parts, including health, work, relationships with family, friends, community and standard of living), reflecting some perceived discrepancy between achievement and an appropriate standard of comparison (Diener *et al.* 1985). The lower the perceived discrepancy, the higher the life satisfaction. As well as achievement, it has been defined in terms of obtaining pleasure from everyday activities, perception of life as meaningful, positive self-image and optimistic outlook (Havighurst 1963; Neugarten *et al.* 1968; Palmore 1979). Sirgy (1998) coined the phrase 'spill-over' model, to explain the association between overall and component assessment (feelings of overall satisfaction may make a person more predisposed to evaluate their standard of living more favourably or vice versa).

The concept is relatively stable, but with some increase in older age (Campbell *et al.* 1976; Campbell 1981) and a decrease in very old age (Bowling *et al.* 1991). The latter may reflect the increased chances of poor health, frailty and life events with very old age. Where satisfaction increases with younger old age, apart from some 'healthy survivor' effects, it may reflect taking on compensatory activities as roles are lost (e.g. with bereavement) (Payne 1988); being able to put one's life context in order (Gatz and Zarit 1999; Blazer 2002); a reluctance to make disapproving self and social evaluations (Schieman 1999); and an increased ability to control exposure or reaction to negative events (Mroczek and Kolarz 1998), which act to maintain well-being (Ryff 1999).

The question of which variables affect life satisfaction is still debated. Most older people report being satisfied with their lives overall, and longitudinal studies have reported that the best predictor of later life satisfaction is earlier life satisfaction (Palmore and Kivett 1977; Palmore *et al.* 1985; Bowling *et al.* 1996), followed by health status, functional ability, mental health, a sense of personal adequacy or usefulness, social networks and activity, and level of income or other indicator of socioeconomic status (but these are all variables which also affect social participation and contacts, which can also affect satisfaction) (Maddox 1963; Lowenthal and Haven 1968; Palmore and Luikart 1972; Markides and Martin 1979; Kushman and Lane 1980; Wenger 1984a; Usui *et al.* 1985; Hayes and Ross 1986; Bowling *et al.* 1991, 1996; Breeze *et al.* 2001). The personality characteristics of extroversion and neuroticism have been reported to account for a moderate amount of the variation detected in perceived well-being and life satisfaction (Costa and McCrae 1984; Costa *et al.* 1987) (see next section on happiness). However, extroversion and neuroticism are highly stable traits, whereas subjective well-being and life satisfaction have only moderate stability, as well as variability, over time (Headey *et al.* 1985; Ehrhardt *et al.* 2000).

Happiness   The other commonly stated indicator of well-being, as well as QoL, is happiness (Sirgy 2002). Most people in affluent societies have been reported to enjoy life, and indicate that they are happy (Veenhoven 1991, 1994; Ehrhardt *et al.* 2000). But what is happiness? Blanchflower and Oswald (2001), following Veenhoven (1991, 1993), defined happiness as QoL – as the degree to which the individual judges the overall quality of his or her life to be favourable or unfavourable. Others have defined happiness (an affective construct) in terms of life satisfaction (a cognitive construct) (Argyle *et al.* 1989). Correlations between measures of these concepts might simply be tapping the underlying factors that the measures have in common (McKennell 1978; Sirgy 2002).

Some investigators have simply taken the concept of happiness at face value. A happiness question has been asked in the US General Social Survey since 1946: 'Taken all together, how would you say things are these days – would you say you are very happy, pretty happy, or not too happy?' (see Gurin *et al.* 1960; Bradburn 1969; Blanchflower and Oswald 2001). This simple item shows stability, and overall, well-being has not risen systematically across time (Blanchflower and Oswald 2001). However, happiness is able to fluctuate on a daily basis (Campbell *et al.* 1976; Andrews and McKennel 1980), in contrast to morale and life satisfaction, which are relatively stable characteristics. It can be divided into two types: hedonic happiness is said to occur with little effort, often as a result of met expectations, whereas effort is crucial to eudemonia which refers to furthering the development of true potential and purpose in life, accompanied by a sense of self-mastery (Scollon and King 2004).

Health has been reported to be the main predictor of both happiness and life satisfaction (Palmore and Luikart 1972; Hayes and Ross 1986; Bowling *et al.*

1996; Michalos *et al.* 2000). Neuroticism is also strongly associated with unhappiness, and extraversion is associated with happiness (Diener and Lucas 2000; Furnham and Petrides 2003).

Morale

Morale is the most poorly defined of all these overlapping concepts, despite its importance in older age (Wenger 1992). Like life satisfaction, it has a cognitive component, which relates to positive/negative feelings (Andrews and McKennel 1980). It has been suggested that it can be measured multi-dimensionally in relation to a person's feelings about their life, himself/herself and their relation to the world (Nydegger 1986). But it is often defined in terms of life satisfaction and acceptance of life, a generalizable feeling of well-being (Lawton 1972, 1975), responses to daily life (Kutner *et al.* 1956), or more specifically as confidence and enthusiasm (George 1979; Stones and Kozma 1980).

A wide range of factors have been linked with morale in older age, particularly social participation and integration, and it is associated with self-image and self-esteem (Blau 1973; Wenger 1992). Changes in life occurring at a greater rate than the perceived average were associated with decreased morale in the Bonn Longitudinal Study of Ageing (Schmitz-Scherzer and Thomae 1983).

Self-esteem and self-concept

Self-esteem is generally defined in terms of self-worth: a belief or evaluation that one is a person of value, accepting personal strengths and weaknesses. It is reflected in one's self-concept or self-image, which can be divided into ideal self (the image they aspire to) and actual self (Coopersmith 1967). Self-concept is also multi-dimensional (e.g. different self-related beliefs can emerge in different life domains – family, friends, romantic relationships, work, standard of living/material (Campbell *et al.* 1976). Both self-esteem and self-concept are important components of emotional well-being, adaptation to ageing (Heidrich and Ryff 1993a; Kling *et al.* 1997), mental health and of life satisfaction (Andrews and Withey 1976a).

It has been proposed that one basis for assessing self-esteem is in terms of the ability to cope with changes in life (Schmitz-Scherzer and Thomae 1983). While there are several commonly used scales of self-esteem in adults of all ages, these are rarely used with older populations (e.g. Fitts 1965; Rosenberg 1965; Coopersmith 1967). In older age, friendship has been reported to be important for promoting self-esteem (Blau 1973). Emler (2001), in his review of the international literature on self-esteem, concluded that those with highest self-esteem were most likely to be risk-takers, and to regard failure to meet their expectations of themselves as 'unlucky'; those with low self-esteem were more likely to commit suicide, to be depressed, lonely, and to be victims of violence and ostracism. Self-esteem has been reported to be positively associated with global life satisfaction (Kozma *et al.* 1991), although this may also reflect shared constructs. Some investigators have regarded self-esteem or self-worth to be 'the linchpin' of QoL for older people, and of adjustment and adaptation in older age (Schwartz 1975; Coleman 1984).

Sense of coherence

Antonovsky (1987) coined the concept of a 'sense of coherence', composed of three elements of comprehensibility, manageability and meaningfulness, defined respectively as:

> a global orientation that expresses the extent to which one has a pervasive, enduring though dynamic, feeling of confidence that (1) the stimuli deriving from one's internal and external environments in the course of living are structured, predictable, and explicable; (2) the resources are available to one to meet the demands posed by these stimuli; and (3) these demands are challenges, worthy of investment and engagement.

These concepts have been little tested, although the inclusion of sense of coherence within a model of quality of life was given some preliminary support in a study of 300 people aged 75+ in Finland (Sarvimäki and Stonbock-Hult 2000).

Social comparisons and expectations theory

Perceived QoL in older age can reflect one's expectations. Social comparisons and gap relativity models encompass past experience, present circumstances and aspirations for the future (Sherif 1936; Hyman 1942; Festinger 1954). Self-assessed status is arguably dependent upon the group one compares oneself with. With this model, QoL is defined as the discrepancy ('gap') between desired and actual circumstances (Krupinski 1980). The key assumption is that people whose life circumstances are closely matched with their aspirations will assess their life as much better than those for whom there is a large gap between actuality and aspirations. Materialists may experience dissatisfaction with their standard of living because they set standard of living goals that are unrealistically high, and because they compare themselves with 'remote', rather than situationally relevant, referents (Sirgy 1998). With this model, indicators aim to capture the individual's achievement of their expectations, hopes and

21

Box 1.4 Types of 'gap theoretical explanation' (Michalos 1986)

- **Goal-achievement gap theory:** satisfaction and happiness are a function of the perceived gap between what one has and what one wants.
- **Ideal-real gap theory:** satisfaction and happiness are a function of the perceived gap between what one has and what is ideal, preferable or desirable.
- **Expectations-reality gap theory:** based on personal likelihood or probability estimates matched against reality.
- **Previous-best comparison theory:** the perceived gap between what one has now and the best one had in the past.
- **Relative deprivation theory:** also known as 'reference class theory' and 'social comparison theory': the gap between what one has and what some relevant other person or group has.
- **Person-environment fit theory or congruence theories:** assessment of the gap between some personal attribute of a person and some aspect of that person's environment.

---

aspirations (Krupinski 1980), in relation to their social comparisons with others (Calman 1984; Michalos 1986; Garratt and Ruta 1999). While innovative attempts have been made to operationalize and measure 'gap' (Garratt and Ruta 1999), there is little supporting evidence of the content validity of the model (see idiographic models, p. 37). Michalos (1986) identified at least six types of 'gap theoretical explanations' in the literature on satisfaction and happiness, and proposed a seventh. These are illustrated in Box 1.4. Michalos' labelled his own gap theory of satisfaction and happiness, based on several hypotheses in combination, as 'multiple discrepancies theory'. By using a combination of three gap theories he was able to explain 45% of the variance in life satisfaction ratings in his own model, and 38% of the variance in happiness, thus making a strong case for his multiple discrepancies theory.

Thus subjective perceptions appear to be homeostatically controlled (Cummins 2000), but few existing models of QoL take people's standards, social comparisons and expectations in life into account. When formulating public policy, it is important to take objective indicators into account when measuring subjective perceptions, in order to avoid the danger of basing services on low public expectations. For example, if someone with low expectations lives in poor-quality housing, they might not necessarily assess its impact on their lives as negatively as someone with higher expectations. The current generation of older people are likely to have low expectations given the challenges and hardships they faced in the first half of the twentieth century. Schieman and Van Gundy (2000), using data from the 1996 and 1998 General Social Surveys in the USA, found that older people reported below average socioeconomic standing than younger people, but they reported greater levels of satisfaction with their income and financial situation (and this then suppressed an increase in depression and distress among older adults). Gap theory, traditionally part of relative deprivation theory, remains controversial.

Psychological theory postulates that while social comparisons may act as mediators to the effects of adverse events and circumstances, and facilitate adaptation to ageing (Heidrich and Ryff 1993b, 1995), they are likely to be only one of several ways in which people cope with life stressors and challenges. Investigators of gap theory also need to take into account other psychological theories, such as perceived level of control over life (Abbey and Andrews 1986). Ryff (1999) suggested three main psychological strategies, including comparisons, for maintaining well-being, and promoting self-mastery and control, in the face of the challenges of ageing: the use of self-enhancing social comparisons (e.g. when in poor health); the development of emotion-focused coping strategies (to control emotional response to situations, including intellectual detachment, denial or reinterpretation of the past) and problem-focused coping strategies aimed at changing or managing the cause of the stress; and psychological centrality, which involves increasing those domains in which one is doing well in order to enhance self-evaluation, and lowering the centrality in which one is not doing well (e.g. losses of health and relationships).

Direction of social comparisons   Social comparisons theory has also been a focal point of analyses of coping behaviour (e.g. among patients) (Taylor *et al.* 1983; Buunk and Gibbons 1998). The direction of the comparison depends upon whether individuals experience positive or negative feelings about their social identity. The lower down the social scale one is, then the opportunities for positive affect decrease and for negative affect increase (Macleod 1999). Thus people state they are more likely to compare upwards when they feel good and downwards when they feel bad (Wheeler and Miyake 1992). This is consistent with the disposition of people who are depressed to engage in negative thoughts (Buunk and Gibbons 1998).

Festingers (1954) earlier hypothesis that people generally choose to compare themselves with superior others has been questioned, and it is now generally believed that such comparisons can be threatening and are usually avoided. People who feel threatened or under stress are believed to compare themselves with others who are *worse off*, which permits individuals to feel better about themselves (Wilson and Benner 1971; Brickman and Bulman 1977). Patients tend to make downward comparisons of themselves with patents worse off than themselves only when experiencing difficulties (Taylor 1983; Michalos 1985; Wood *et al.* 1985, Affleck 1987; De Vellis *et al.* 1990), and make upward comparisons with people healthier than themselves when setting standards for their recovery and performance (Blalock *et al.* 1989, 1990).

This theory is likely to be relevant to older populations who are vulnerable to social exclusion due to ageist attitudes in society, lower incomes, reduced levels of independence and often sub-optimal access to preventive and specialist services (Bowling 1999; Hill *et al.* 1999). Mechanic and Angel (1987), on the basis of their survey of 2431 Americans, reported that older people's evaluations of their health were not absolute, but relative, and made in the context of social comparisons. Farquhar (1995) reported, on the basis of her qualitative interviews with older people in East London and Essex, that people frequently referred to others who were worse off than them when evaluating their own QoL. Downward comparisons would be expected among this generation of older people, who lived through a major depression, a world war, food rationing, and had no entitlement to universal health care free at the point of use until 1948, and emphasize the need to measure both objective and subjective indicators of QoL.

Optimism and pessimism

Optimism is a personality construct. Dispositional optimism refers to generalized outcome expectancies that good, rather than bad, things will happen. Situational optimism refers to the positive or negative expectations of an individual for a specific situation. Pessimism refers to the reverse tendency to expect the worst. Both types of optimism are stable dispositional resources that influence whether a person will be able to remain focused on reducing discrepancies between behaviour and aspirations (Carver and Scheier 1981).

Dispositional optimism has been reported to correlate fairly highly with self-mastery, trait anxiety, neuroticism and self-esteem (Scheier *et al.* 1994). In contrast to pessimism, it has been reported to be positively correlated with reduced levels of hostility and depression, use of denial as a coping mechanism, post-surgical self-rated QoL and faster recovery (Scheier *et al.* 1989). This may partly explain why people with serious disabilities often report their QoL to be good (Albrecht and Devlieger 1999). Optimists apparently do better at work, suffer less from depression, respond better to stress and, possibly by boosts to their immune system, have lower morbidity and mortality rates. Optimism is central to coping, adjustment and mental health (Pearlin and Schooler 1978; Gatz and Zarit 1999). It benefits people when they are adjusting to deteriorating health or other changing circumstances, and may thus lead to perceptions of higher QoL (Diener *et al.* 1991; Sprangers and Schwartz 1999). Accommodative coping, in which one adjusts one's goals to take account of situational constraints, and which is essential to 'successful ageing' (Baltes and Baltes 1990b; Fry 2000), is related to optimism in older age (Brandstadler and Renner 1990; Blazer 2002).

Optimism and risk perception   Weinstein (1980) reported that most people are optimists and tend to underestimate their risks, or vulnerability, to negative events, including health events. It is believed that self-risk assessments are influenced by downward social comparisons with worse-off others (i.e. those who are perceived to be more vulnerable), with the effect of leading the individual to feel less vulnerable (Buunk and Gibbons 1998). Older people are regarded as 'optimists' and 'health optimists' overall. It has long been documented that, in older old age, people tend to rate their lives as the same or better than younger elderly people, and more favourably than their doctors rated them (Suchman and Phillips 1958; Andrews and Withey 1976a; Campbell *et al.* 1976). They are more likely than younger people to adapt or modify their expectations (Thomas 1981), and to react defensively and deny unpleasant or anxiety-provoking facts, particularly those outside their control (Tobin and Lieberman 1976). But other research reports that adults of all ages overestimate their risks in specific situations (Sutton 1998). For example, the public is generally unrealistic about the level of crime (Dodd *et al.* 2004), and older people often feel personally vulnerable and fear crime, although the chances of burglary in England and Wales are relatively low in households whose head is aged 65 or over (Home Office 2000). Walker and Walker (2005) suggested that older people's unrealistic perceptions of their risks of becoming crime victims may reflect the longer time it takes them to recover from injuries, and their reduced physical ability to escape from attackers.

Self-efficacy, self-mastery, autonomy and control

Self-efficacy, or mastery, is a personality construct, and refers to one's competency and capability of success in producing an intended goal. It is the ability to maintain some control over life, and the ability to preserve a sense of control

25

in the face of the changes which can accompany ageing (Blazer 2002). It is a key to successful ageing (Baltes and Baltes 1990b). In theory, an individual's cognitive beliefs and expectations about their self-efficacy, mastery or ability are related to their motivations and actions (Bandura 1977). The extent to which people perceive that they, rather than others, determine what happens in their lives leads to a greater sense of internal control (Lefcourt 1982), which leads to greater self-esteem and greater perceived self-efficacy, which influences intentions, coping, behaviour and ultimately well-being (Mirowsky and Ross 1991; Pearlin 1999; Eckenrode and Hamilton 2000). These concepts are generally included within models of successful ageing (Larson 1978; Grundy and Bowling 1999; Bowling et al. 2003).

Evidence indicates that levels of perceived control increase during early adulthood, peak during middle age and are lower among older adults (Gecas 1989), leaving older people potentially more vulnerable. Control over life, self-efficacy, self-sufficiency, independence (freedom from control in function, action, judgement), and autonomy (the freedom to determine one's own actions, free from controlling influences) can be important for maintenance of good life quality in older age (Abbey and Andrews 1986; Abeles 1991; Lawton 1991; Liberman 1991; Wetle 1991; Perrig-Chiello 1999). Studies of middle-aged and older people have documented their emphasis on maintaining their independence, on being able to carry out their daily activities and look after themselves. Even iller respondents are apparently able to perceive themselves as independent if support services facilitate them in maintaining their physical independence at home (Hayden et al. 1999). Control over daily life is one of older people's priorities as an outcome indicator of social care (Netten et al. 2002).

Older age is a time where freedom of choice may be at risk of being constrained by reduced finances as a result of retirement from paid work (although this can also bring new freedoms from routine responsibilities). Personal freedom to continue with routine activities of daily living and social activities may be reduced by frailty and functional limitations, leading to risk of dependency. Each of these freedoms is particularly threatened for frail older people, and those who give up their homes and environmental identities and move into institutionalized care settings (Clark and Bowling 1989, 1990; Abeles 1991; Lawton 1991; Liberman 1991; Wetle 1991). But even those who live in institutions can be enabled to make autonomous choices and state preferences. The importance of perceived control to people is also evident in other areas (e.g. among people with health problems) (Devins and Seland 1987; see also Blazer 2002).

Opportunities for self-actualization and development may be facilitated or inhibited by the structure of wider society. While older people might enjoy the greater freedom that retirement from paid work can bring, level of income (also affected by public policies) and level of personal- or agency-led social and practical support can enable or inhibit participation, autonomy and self-actualization. The social capital, perceived safety and access to facilities within an area are all factors that might affect both autonomy and self-actualization. Discrimination may be experienced by older age groups and can inhibit social participation as well as restrict access to appropriate services (Bowling 1999; Bowling et al. 2001; Seshamani and Gray 2002). Thus a sense of self-efficacy is not solely dependent on cognitive factors. However, there is also debate about whether self-efficacy is a causal or mediating variable of subjective QoL.

Mediating variables

Some concepts commonly applied to QoL have potential roles as influences, constituents or mediators of perceived life quality. Distinguishing between these different types of variable may lead to more appropriate measurement scales (Zizzi et al. 1998; Fayers and Hand 2002). The effects of personality on perceived well-being and QoL are controversial, partly because of the debate about causal vs. mediating variables. The distinction between what aspects of QoL are 'staits' or 'traits' is also unclear (Joyce et al. 1999). Extroversion and neuroticism have been reported to account for a moderate amount of the variation in subjective well-being (Costa et al. 1987; Spiro and Bossé 2000), although these associations have been contested (Headey et al. 1985). There is also a strong body of literature suggesting a link between psychological variables (e.g. depression, hopelessness or pessimism) and ill-health, including mortality (Engel 1968; Stansfeld et al. 2002). However, interpretations of such data are complex because of the process of adaptation and the buffering effects of potential mediating variables (Brickman and Campbell 1971). Research on the effect of psychological variables has been limited largely to the literature on patients with diagnosed mental health problems or college students (Rosenfield 1992, 1989; Mercier and King 1993; Zizzi et al. 1998).

Despite classic work on mediating variables in the 1980s, theoretical and empirical development has made little progress. Abbey and Andrews (1986) developed a conceptual model based on the assumption that people's interactions with their social world influenced their social-psychological make-up, and in turn influenced their own internal states of depression and anxiety.

Following Abbey and Andrews (1985), Barry (1997) and Zizzi et al. (1998) argued that there is a need for a model of QoL which focuses on the link between psychological factors and subjective evaluations of QoL. They indicated that subjectively perceived QoL is *mediated* by several interrelated variables, including self-related constructs (e.g. self-mastery and self-efficacy, morale and self-esteem, perceived control/mastery over life), and these perceptions are *influenced* by cognitive mechanisms (e.g. expectations of life, social values, beliefs, aspirations and social comparison standards) (Zizzi et al. 1998).

Health and functioning models

Perceived health is a significant part of HRQoL and QoL (see Bowling 2001, 2004a). Descartes ([1637] 1953) asserted that health is the highest good; its preservation is the first good, and the foundation of all other goods in life. It is a direct component of well-being and contributes to a person's basic ability to function in their social roles, to pursue valued activities and goals in life and to choose the life which they value (Sen 1985; Anand 2002). It is a 'special good', which also justifies the case for egalitarianism in health because inequalities in health result in inequalities in a person's capability to function and in their freedom (Berlin 1969; Anand 2002). Health is certainly important to people. In a national population survey of the most important areas of life, one's own health was self-nominated by about four in ten of all adult respondents, and by almost two thirds of those aged 65 and over (most commonly nominated by these respondents as the first most important area, but most commonly prioritized after relationships among younger respondents) (Bowling 1995a, 1995b, 1996). As might be expected, those who had lost their health were most likely to prioritize this as the most important area of life. This is consistent with gap theory, that people value what they have lost or aspire to (Michalos 1986). Although the direction of associations is not always known, good levels of physical and mental functioning and general health status have long been associated with perceived well-being, morale and overall quality of life (Zautra and Hempel 1984; Wood 1987; Burholt 2001; Michalos et al. 2001), and the associations have been replicated in large surveys (Bowling 1995a, 1995b; Bowling et al. 1996, 1999; Bowling and Windsor 2001; Breeze et al. 2001).

Common diseases in older age are diseases of the cardiovascular, respiratory and musculoskeletal systems. Other chronic diseases of older age include mental conditions (depression and dementia) and sensory impairments; and common problems among frail, older people relate to mobility, balance, vision and hearing. For example, in Britain, the most commonly reported causes of long-standing illness, disability and infirmity among people aged 65 and over are disorders of the musculoskeletal system (particularly among women), and the heart and circulatory system, followed by respiratory disorders, endocrine and metabolic conditions and digestive conditions (Bridgwood 2000). However, most older people consider their health to be good, although those in the lower socioeconomic groups are less likely to rate their health positively (Browne *et al.* 1994; Nybo *et al.* 2001; Marmot *et al.* 2003). People living in nursing or care homes, and those with dementia, are often excluded from population surveys. Given the increasing prevalence of dementia among older people, its neglect has left gaps in the body of knowledge of QoL in older age.

The evidence on risk, and on the plasticity of ageing processes, within limits, suggests that theories of homeostasis require some modification (Brouwer 1990; Grundy 2001). As Grundy pointed out, while the risk of developing Alzheimer's disease increases markedly with age, most older people do not develop this condition. Again, while functional decline is associated with increasing old age, regular aerobic exercise has been reported to increase the maximal aerobic power in women aged over 79 (Malbut *et al.* 2002; see also editorial by Greig 2002), and strength training can improve muscle strength and physical functioning (McMurdo 2000). Health behaviour can influence health status and new roles and activities can be started. But, as Grundy (2001) also argued, it is often difficult to begin to accumulate reserves in older age.

The concept of HRQoL has also been based on the 'pathology' 'dis-ease' model of ill-health and dependency, referred to earlier, and has focused on the negative impact on life of (ill-)health status and 'dis-ease' (McKevitt *et al.* 2002). The emphasis has been on (dys)functional status (the level of ability to perform socially allocated roles free of physical or mental health-related limitations – Bowling 2004a). Functionalism underpins this approach, with its focus on ability and role performance, essential to the continuing functioning of the wider society. The aim of measurement has usually been to track the speed of return to normal activities (Scheir *et al.* 1989). The World Health Organization (WHO) has attempted to redress the balance away from dis-ability and towards ability models of health and HRQoL outcomes. This is reflected in the shift of focus from its *International Classification of Impairments, Disabilities and Handicaps* (World Health Organization 1980), which distinguished between physical status (impairment), physical functioning (disability) and social functioning (handicap) and towards its more positive *International Classification of Impairments* (of 'structure'), *Activities* (formerly called disabilities) *and Participation* (formerly called handicaps)

(World Health Organization 1998), and its components of health classification, known as the *International Classification of Functioning, Disability and Health* (World Health Organization 2001). The WHO's (1948) earlier definition of health 'as a state of complete physical, mental and social well-being' appears to act as the lead for the measurement of QoL as an indicator of health and social care outcomes. While Utopian, it has generated broader measures of health which incorporate social, physical and psychological well-being, rather than sole reliance on traditional indicators based on prevalence of risk factors, chronic conditions and mortality rates. This, in turn, accentuated the interest in the broader concept of QoL, or HRQoL, in health outcomes research. However, the broadest indicators of life quality, ranging from subjective indicators of life satisfaction and happiness to objective indicators of income, environmental and community resources, are regarded as less relevant to the goals of health care interventions (Patrick and Erickson 1993).

The conceptual and measurement confusion surrounding HRQoL is evident in the multitude of different measurement scales used to tap it. Garratt *et al.*'s (2002) systematic review of the literature on patient-assessed health status and QoL was based on a multi-dimensional classification (Sanders *et al.* 1998) that included:

- dimension-specific measures (e.g. psychological well-being measured using an anxiety and/or depression scale such as the General Health Questionnaire – Goldberg and Williams 1988);

- disease- or population-specific measures, which may be multi-domain, relevant to specific health problems (e.g. the Asthma Quality of Life Questionnaire – Juniper *et al.* 1993);

- generic measures which can be used across population types, usually multi-domain measures of broader health status (e.g. the Short-Form 36 Health Survey (SF-36 – Ware and Sherbourne 1992);

- individualized measures which enable respondents to nominate and weight important areas of their own life (e.g. the Schedule for Evaluation of Individual Quality of Life – Hickey *et al.* 1999 – or the Patient-Generated Index – Garratt and Ruta 1999);

- utility measures which incorporate preferences for health states, in order to produce a single index used for making comparisons across treatments and between health problems for economic evaluation (e.g. the EuroQoL – EuroQoL Group 1990 – and the Health Utilities Index – Feeny *et al.* 1995).

They reported finding 23,042 records (articles) after removal of duplicates, published during 1990–9. Although there was evidence of the use of a small number of generic measures suggesting a standardized approach, among disease-specific measures there was little standardization.

Social health, social networks, support and activity

The largest body of empirical research on the various facets of well-being has focused on the structure, functioning and supportiveness of human relationships, the social context in which people live and integration within society. Some investigators use the term 'social capital' to embrace both the characteristics of individuals' personal relationships and support structures, and their access to enabling community resources, although others use it to encompass only the latter.

An emphasis on social health in investigations of well-being and QoL is supported by research on the public's priorities in life. In the survey mentioned earlier of the most important things in life, just over half of all adult respondents self-nominated relationships, and a fifth nominated social life and leisure activities; about half of those aged 65+ nominated relationships (most commonly ranked second in importance after health; in contrast younger respondents most commonly ranked relationships as most important) and about a fifth nominated social life and leisure activities (Bowling 1996; Bowling and Windsor 2001). Social relationships, contacts and activities were nominated by people aged 65 and over as highly important to their QoL in other studies (Browne *et al.* 1994; Farquhar 1995).

Parsons (1951) pointed out that society's expectations and social norms concerning individuals' roles and behaviour had effects on their health. Dubos (1959) also long ago argued that health cannot be defined in isolation of social communities and must be seen in terms of the ability of individuals to function in a manner acceptable to themselves and their social groups. Thus, Donald *et al.* (1978), following Caplan (1974) and Cassel (1976), conceptualized social health as the social support system that might intervene and modify the effect of the environment and stress on both mental and physical health. In their definition, the measurement of social health focuses on the individual, defined by interpersonal interactions and social participation and activity; both objective constructs and subjective evaluations were included. Additional areas of social health include personal and work achievements, position in the hierarchy and sexual satisfaction (Kaplan 1975).

31

Social networks are the social relationships that surround a person, their characteristics and individuals' perceptions and valuations of them. Network characteristics include their size, density (connectedness between members), boundedness (e.g. by neighbourhood), homogeneity, frequency of contact of members, their multiplexity (number of types of transactions within them), duration and reciprocity (Berkman and Glass 2000). Social support is the interactive process in which emotional, instrumental or financial aid is obtained from network members. Lack of social integration and social support can decrease the individual's resources for dealing with social stress, and has been implicated in poor mental health outcomes (George et al. 1989). The importance of social networks, and their characteristics, then, lies in the extent to which they fulfil members' needs (Walker et al. 1997).

Research interest in social support was revitalized in the 1970s by Caplan (1974), Cassel (1976), Cobb (1976) and Kaplan et al. (1977). It was believed that social support maintained the organism by promoting adaptive behaviour or neuroendocrine responses when under stress, or in receipt of other threats to health. Much of the literature indicates that social relationships and activity per se appear to confer health benefits through psychosocial pathways. A meta-analysis of the literature on social support from 1970 to 1998 showed that social relationships can act to promote health as well as lead to worse health outcomes, requiring a greater recognition in research of both the positive and negative elements in relationships (Seeman 2000). The research evidence strongly supports an association between poor social support and increased risk of mortality in vulnerable groups of people, such as the widowed, and elderly people living in institutions, although intervening variables which might explain associations have often been inadequately controlled for (see review by Bowling and Grundy 1998). There is also strong evidence, support-ed by longitudinal research, that lack of social support contributes to coronary heart disease morbidity and mortality in men (Berkman and Syme 1979; Ruberman et al. 1984; Berkman et al. 1992; see also reviews by Olsen 1992 and Bowling and Grundy 1998), although the evidence is unclear for women. Even owning pets has been reported to influence positively well-being and survival, although the research is also inconsistent (Friedmann and Thomas 1995; Beck and Meyers 1996; Raina et al. 1999).

Social support has also been reported to be associated with proxy measures of QoL such as life satisfaction, morale and well-being (Breeze et al. 2001). Social participation, activity and having friends, particularly a confidant, is important for maintenance of morale and self-esteem, feeling loved, security, autonomous self-image, self-mastery, prevention of loneliness, well-being and mental health, especially if relationships are reciprocal (Lowenthal and Haven 1968; Blau 1973; Brown and Harris 1978; Lawton 1980; Wentowski 1981; Bowling 1991, 1994; Wenger 1992; Victor *et al.* 2000; Bowling *et al.* 2002a; Silverstein and Parker 2002). It is still unknown whether social support has a direct effect on health and well-being, for example by providing comfort, feedback or practical help which reduces symptoms or stressors, whether support disturbs or mitigates the relationship between stress and health (Holahan and Moos 1981), or whether lack of support leads to psychological damage (see reviews by Bowling 1991, 1994). But health and mobility are also essential for maintaining independence, social contacts and participation (Jylhä 2001), and physical health status and functional ability are stronger predictors of life satisfaction in older age than social network and support structure (Bowling and Browne 1991; Bowling *et al.* 1996).

A large amount of research literature exists on the structure and functioning of people's relationships. People attain older age with the support network they have built up over a lifetime, although there are differences by social group. People without children have higher proportions of siblings, friends and neighbours in their networks, and single women compensate for relatives by maintaining strong contacts with friends (Wenger *et al.* 2000). Women also report more friends than men, with men being more likely to rely on wives for intimacy and friendship, and people in lower socioeconomic groups report weaker friendship ties but stronger links with kin. People who are more highly educated have more friends and fewer relatives in their networks (Wenger 1996).

Some research indicates that older people report fewer conflictual social relationships (which may adversely affect well-being) than younger people (Schieman and Van Gundy 2000). It has been suggested that this is because older age is accompanied by a maturity, greater knowledge, growing insight and sense of others, and skill at handling disharmony (Mirowsky and Ross 1992). On the other hand, older people may report fewer emotions that entail disapproving self evaluations and social evaluations (Schieman 1999). The increased risks of widow(er)hood with older age, and the number of people without children, emphasizes the importance of maintenance of wider social networks in older age (Bowling and Cartwright 1982; Bowling and Windsor 1995; Cotton 1999).

Apparently, networks composed largely of relatives are more effective at providing instrumental help (Wenger 1989; Wenger and Shahtahmasebi 1990; Rettig and Leichtentritt 1999). While high-density networks, where members know each other, might increase the potential for conflict between members, their members are also the most likely to provide help in emergencies (see review by Bowling 1994). Friends are also essential for companionship, emotional support, morale and reducing feelings of loneliness among older people. Provision of a wider range of resources (emotional support, practical help, advice and companionship) is highest in networks composed of both relatives *and* friends (Bowling and Grundy 1998). Social support and network sizes are also dynamic, and can be negative or positive in effect (Wentowski 1981; Bowling *et al.* 1995a, 1995b); and networks composed of more friends or neighbours than relatives are more changeable (e.g. ties weaken). Their size may depend on cultural, personality, situational and neighbourhood characteristics, and opportunities to access available communication systems (whether by telephone, use of transport, physical mobility or email and mobile phone networks).

Given that the characteristics of the neighbourhood can constrain friendships and involvement in social activities, neighbourhood is also theoretically associated with the well-being of older people (Lawton 1980; Berkman and Glass 2000) (see next section).

Social cohesion and social capital

Human ecology theory holds that the QoL of humans and the quality of their environment are interdependent (Rettig and Leichtentritt 1999). Social scientists have long focused on why some communities prosper and benefit their citizens, and others do not, focusing mainly on social inequalities (Wilkinson 1996). Social cohesion and social capital are collective, ecological dimensions of society, distinct from the concepts of social networks and social support which are measured only at the individual level (Kawachi and Berkman 2000). Durkheim ([1895] 1982, [1897] 1997) recognized long ago that well-being is influenced by society as a whole. Therefore in order to understand individuals we must study them in the context of external, societal as well as internal, personal forces. This is the reasoning behind many social regeneration programmes (Pilkington 2002; Watkins *et al.* 2002).

The definition and measurement of social capital are still evolving. Most definitions reflect an uneasy conceptual mix of community membership (structure) and moral resources of trust and reciprocity. It is typically measured with questions about group membership, social, civic and political participation, and feelings of trust, social cohesion or communality with the neighbourhood as well as the characteristics of social relationships and participation (Cooper *et al.* 1999). Objective indicators include crime rates, access to shopping, leisure and sports facilities, areas of scenic quality and housing type (Flax 1972; Rogerson *et al.* 1989a, 1989b; Rogerson 1995). Subjective indicators include levels of area satisfaction and perceptions of neighbourliness and safety (Rogerson *et al.* 1989a, 1989b; Cooper *et al.* 1999). The special signifi-cance of historical and present attachment to place of residence among older people is also beginning to be explored (Rubinstein and Parmelee 1992), although residential satisfaction is reportedly unrelated to the proximity of community resources among older populations (see Kahana *et al.* 2003).

A socially cohesive society is marked by its supportiveness, shared value systems and identities, connectiveness, a sense of belonging, solidarity between groups, trust and reciprocity (Kawachi and Berkman 2000), rather than forcing individuals to rely entirely on their own resources (Durkheim [1897] 1997), and is well endowed with stocks of social capital (Kawachi and Berkman 2000). It is typically measured with questions about feelings of commitment and trust, values and norms and feelings of belonging. Social capital is a subset of the concept of social cohesion. It refers to the extent to which communities offer members opportunities and resources – through active involvement in social activities, voluntary work, group membership, leisure and recreation facilities, political activism and educational facilities – to increase their *personal* resources (Coleman 1988; Putnam 1995; Brissette *et al.* 2000; Kawachi and Berkman 2000). Putnam (1995) defined social capital in terms of connections among individuals, social networks and the norms of reciprocity and trust that they create, and in terms of the characteristics of organizations which facilitate beneficial cooperation and organization between members. Putnam suggested that social capital is in decline; the action required to stem this involves designing communities which encourage interpersonal interaction, and to promote social connections with others, rather than solitary activities. In this context, society's undervaluation of older people needs addressing (Boaz *et al.* 1999; Pfizer 2002).

Neighbourhood disadvantage (e.g. by repeated exposure to stressful and threatening conditions) is likely to have a negative impact on health. High levels of social capital have been reported to be independently associated with lower mortality rates and also with better self-rated health and functional sta-tus (Kawachi *et al.* 1997a, 1997b, 1999; Kawachi and Berkman 2000; Ross and Mirowsky 2001). Lawton (1980) also reported that the quality of the neigh-bourhood can influence the emotional well-being of older people. Grundy and Bowling (1999) analysed features of the neighbourhood in their analyses of the QoL of 630 people aged 85+ living at home. Whether respondents liked the area their lived in, whether they felt anxiety or fear about intruders, going out or opening the door at home, and whether their homes were warm enough for them were among nine variables which distinguished between those respondents with a good or poor QoL. The inadequacy and expense of public transport and perceived fears for safety while travelling are also potential barriers to retaining independence among older people (Hayden *et al.* 1999; Marmot *et al.* 2003). As Walker and Walker (2005) have discussed, access to transport is an even bigger problem for older people who live in rural areas. Studies have reported an association between the independence that car ownership gives, access to good public transport, and higher perceived QoL (Webster *et al.* 2002; Gilhooley *et al.* 2003). The need for improved reliability of public transport, improvements to perceived safety and security, more public transport that caters for the needs of those with health problems, and guidance for older drivers, are all relevant (Department of Transport 2000).

Environmental contexts

Environmental gerontology, which examines the relation between elderly persons and their sociospatial surroundings (Wahl and Weisman 2003), or 'ageing in place' (Gitlin 2003), is increasingly important. The design of enabling internal and external environments can promote the independence, social participation and QoL of older people (Schaie *et al.* 2003). Research on residential care environments has informed community care policies in relation to 'age-friendly' societies (Kendig 2003), although better information is still required which describes 'how individuals use, manipulate, or perform tasks in their settings' (Golant 2003).

Despite the importance of understanding ageing in one's home environment, most research in this area is descriptive and lacks theoretical direction (Gitlin 2003). With policy and societal interest in active ageing, it is especially important to focus on the fit between the individual and his or her surroundings for the promotion of independence and well-being in later life (Wahl 2001; Iwarsson 2003; Schaie *et al.* 2003; Wahl *et al.* 2003). Associations have been reported between housing technology (even access to dish-washers) and life satisfaction among older people (Wahl and Mollenkopf 2003). It is expected that interest in new technologies will increase (Peeters *et al.* 2001). Technological innovations can be divided into those which facilitate everyday tasks, enhance safety (including monitoring links), compensate for sensory and mobility losses (including communication links), and rehabilitative and nursing technologies which aim to enhance independence (see Weidekamp-Maicher 2001).

A contemporary model of QoL in older age needs to incorporate aspects of twenty-first-century life, such as access to, and opportunity to take advantage of (e.g. through education, income levels, costs, availability), new technologies (Sixsmith and Sixsmith 2001). And access to essential facilities should not be overlooked: lifts in blocks of flats that work, effective central heating, and so on. QoL is dependent upon having the opportunity to aim for, and achieve, personal goals, as well as access to the economic, personal, environmental and community resources to facilitate this.

Multi-dimensionality and global assessment of QoL

A global QoL assessment (e.g. 'How do you rate the quality of your life as a whole?') is an individual's overall evaluation of a wide range of complex, diverse and potentially interacting physical, psychological, social, economic, community and societal considerations. Definitions of QoL tend to focus on this multi-dimensionality. Beckie and Hayduk (1997) and Fayers and Hand (2002) argued that such definitions confound the dimensionality of the concept with the multiplicity of the causal sources of QoL. Beckie and Hayduk (1997) pointed out that QoL could be considered as a global personal assessment of a single dimension which may be causally responsive to a variety of other distinct dimensions: it is a unidimensional concept with multiple causes. They argued that it is thus logical for a unidimensional indicator of QoL (e.g. a self-rating global QoL uniscale) to be the dependent variable in analyses, and the predictor variables include the range of health, social and psychological variables. As the authors pointed out, this can be problematic for causal analyses if the QoL evaluation is greater than the sum of its parts, but the diversity, multiplicity and complexity of sources of QoL warrants treating its measurement in terms of a global assessment. This whole debate is still inconclusive.

Idiographic models

Recognition of the need for broader definitions of QoL, taking individuals' perceptions into account, has resulted in the wider adoption of the WHO Quality of Life Group's (WHOQOL Group 1993) definition of QoL as a person's perception of life, in the context of their culture, value systems, goals, expectations, standards and concerns, as affected by their physical health, psychological state, independence, social relationships and environment. But

37

a single scale rarely covers all these areas adequately, and individual-level perceptions are, in any case, lost in group analyses (Bowling 1995a). Even the 100-item WHOQOL Group's measure of QoL (WHOQOL Group 1993; Skevington 1999; Skevington *et al.* 1999) fails to provide adequate feedback.

While there are more attempts to base social indicators on social theory (Walker 2002, 2005), lay theories are equally important. In contrast to the large body of quantitative research, phenomenological perspectives hold that QoL is a subjective concept, which is dependent upon the interpretations and perceptions of the individual (Ziller 1974). This is referred to as an individualized or idiographic approach. It could be argued that human beings strive for meaning and towards a goal of self-actualization, and therefore a phenomenological perspective is appropriate (Campbell 1972; O'Boyle 1997). QoL, from this perspective, is not measurable in a standardized way.

Thus while the division of QoL into pre-defined individual components (e.g. physical, psychological and social functioning) is helpful for measurement purposes, this approach may not tap the most pertinent domains of people's perceptions of QoL, or their subjectivity. The increasing focus on psychometric abilities in scale development, and the constant search for shorter measurement scales, carries the risk that areas of importance to large numbers of the populations of interest are omitted from questionnaires if they fail to 'perform'. Idiographic or individualized, hermeneutic approaches use semistructured interview techniques (Browne *et al.* 1994; O'Boyle 1997; Garratt and Ruta 1999; Hickey *et al.* 1999). But a tension remains between objective and subjective approaches to the conceptualization and measurement of QoL. This mirrors the tension which is often apparent between qualitative and quantitative social researchers, with only a few seeking to utilize both methods to complement each other, rather than perceiving them to be irretrievably, theoretically and conceptually opposed.

When lay people have not been consulted in the development of a questionnaire, then the items within it will reflect the values and assumptions held by 'experts', and research results will not necessarily reflect the perspectives of respondents (Fox-Rushby and Parker 1995). Where research on people's concepts of QoL has involved asking them to prioritize areas of life from a predefined list, then the concepts will again reflect the views of the 'experts' (Fernàndez-Ballesteros 1993). Moreover, the negative focus of most existing questionnaires carries the danger of under-emphasizing good QoL. Interviews with older people show that they emphasize both good and bad aspects of life quality (Nilsson *et al.* 1998).

Overlap between theoretical and lay models

So what is the overlap between theoretical and lay models of QoL? Juniper *et al.* (1997) compared two philosophically different methods for selecting items for a disease-specific QoL questionnaire: the impact method which selects items that are most frequently perceived as important by patients (albeit from a pre-prepared list of 152 items from the literature and consultations with professionals, but not patients), and the psychometric method (factor analysis) which selects items primarily according to their relationships with one another. They reported, from their research on adult asthma patients, that the impact method resulted in a 32-item instrument and the psychometric method led to a 36-item tool, with 20 items common to both. The psychometric approach had discarded the items relating to emotional function and environment, and included items mainly on fatigue instead. Thus the two approaches led to important differences. Kane *et al.* (1998), in a comparative study of the USA and Europe, compared geriatric professionals' and lay people's ratings of the importance of 32 items measuring physical functioning. While the overall correlation between the groups was 0.82, in general lay people rated instrumental activities of daily living items more highly in importance (e.g. (dis-)ability to prepare meals, clean the house, shopping). The experts rated the most dysfunctional activities of daily living items higher in importance than the lay people (e.g. (dis-)ability to dress, feed self, get to/use toilet).

The need for measures of QoL to be more sensitive to differing values, and changes in priorities with increasing age, is supported by research reporting that people aged 75 and over were more likely than younger respondents to prioritize their own health, and the ability to get out and about, and were less likely to prioritize social relationships, finances and work. Women of all ages were also more likely than men to prioritize social relationships, and men were more likely than women to prioritize finances; respondents in the lowest social classes were more likely than other respondents to prioritize their own health and they were less likely to prioritize social relationships (Bowling 1995a, 1995b). Differing priorities present a challenge not only to the design and content validity of QoL measures, but also to their scoring and/or weighting. If measurement scales give equal weighting to their various sub-domains, it is unlikely that the domains will have equal significance to different social groups and individuals within these. Even where scales are weighted it is unlikely that the weightings will be equally applicable to different groups and individuals. Moreover, methodology literature comparing standardized weighted and unweighted cardinal (i.e. summed) scales has consistently reported no benefits of more complex weighted methods in relation to the proportion of explained variance or sensitivity to change over time (Andrews and Crandall 1976; Headey and Wearing 1989; Jenkinson et al. 1991).

O'Boyle (1997) agued that, given the heterogeneity of the elderly population, it is unlikely that any single measure will be suitable for all purposes. His measure of quality of life – the Schedule for Evaluation of Individual Quality of Life (SEIQoL) conceptualizes QoL as whatever the individual determines it to be (Hickey et al. 1999). It measures the areas of life that are important to the respondent, how people rate themselves in each area and the relative importance of the areas. It is still unclear, however, which of the individualized instruments is most reliable and valid, and how they fully compare with standardized methods (Fitzpatrick 1999).

Groups are made up of individuals, and group statistics inevitably sacrifice individual-level information. The content validity of existing standardized measures requires addressing if meaningful measurement is to be achieved (Joyce et al. 1999). But while different social groups, and individuals, prioritize different areas of life (Browne et al. 1994; Bowling 1995a, 1995b; Scharf and Smith 2003; Nazroo et al. 2004), there is evidence from the same studies that a shared core of common values also exists. The author's research, presented in this book, was based on both quantitative and qualitative approaches (Bowling et al. 2002a, 2003; Bowling and Gabriel 2004; Gabriel and Bowling 2004a, 2004b). It found that measures of QoL based on the theoretical literature largely overlapped with older people's own perceptions of QoL, but with important exceptions. The central drivers of QoL, which were consistently emphasized by all methods, were psychological mechanisms (e.g. psychological outlook, optimism-pessimism), health and functional status, personal social networks, support and activities, and neighbourhood social capital. However, in contrast to the quantitative models of influences on self-rated QoL, the lay models also emphasized the importance of financial circumstances and independence, which need to be incorporated into a definition of broader QoL. This is supported by a more recent systematic review of the literature of the components of QoL nominated by older people themselves, reported on in 42 distinct studies (Brown et al. 2004). It was reported that these were remarkably consistent and covered the following broad themes as important to older people for their QoL: social relationships; social and leisure activities; quality of the neighbourhood; emotional well-being; religion and spirituality; independence; mobility; autonomy; finances and standard of living; health and the health of others. The studies held on the World Database of Happiness also indicate, directly or indirectly, that most people value health, wealth, security, knowledge, freedom, honesty and equality as contributors to well-being (Veenhoven 1996, 1997; Heylighen and Bernheim 2000).

Integrated, composite models

Conceptualizations and indicators of QoL have included a wide range of domains (e.g. Arnold 1991), but they have usually been separated rather than presented as comprehensive, whole or interlinked areas. Grundy and Bowling (1999) attempted to develop a composite model of QoL and to identify the oldest old with a cumulatively very good and very poor QoL. They defined QoL on the basis of the literature and focus group research on what gave older people's lives quality and what took it away. Their final factor model incorporated and represented four life domains: autonomy and perceived well-being; environment; mental and physical health and functioning; and social activities. These variables distinguished between older people participating in a census of 660 people aged 85+ in East London, on a continuum of the composite measure (e.g. 58% of men and 41% of women achieved 'good' scores on at least five of the nine indicators of QoL used). Von Faber *et al.* (2001) also attempted a composite measure of 'successful ageing' in their study (census) of 599 people aged 85 and over living in Leiden. They judged respondents to be 'successfully aged' (defined as 'a state of being') if they achieved optimal scores on each indicator used of physical, social and psychocognitive functioning (but only 10% of respondents achieved optimal scores, suggesting that their non-continuum approach was too narrow).

Fry (2000) attempted an integrational framework to investigate the concept of QoL in older age, using a (non-random) postal survey of 465 households in Vancouver and Victoria, British Columbia, and in-depth interviews with a sub-sample of respondents. The themes which emerged from the analysis of the in-depth interviews corresponded well with those which emerged from the questionnaire data. The authors concluded that their findings showed that older adults valued personal control, autonomy and self-sufficiency, their right to pursue a chosen lifestyle and a right to privacy. Thus, the use of multiple methods played an important role.

Conclusion

QoL, then, is inherently a dynamic, multi-level and complex concept, reflecting objective, subjective, macro-societal and micro-individual, positive and

41

negative influences which interact together (Lawton 1991). A life-course perspective is also required, as a person's reserve in later life reflects a lifetime's accumulation, and depletion, of resources and skills (Grundy 2001). But there is no still agreement on definitions, which poses inevitable challenges for measurement. The literature reveals that QoL, while reflecting common core values, can still encompass a wide ranging array of domains. There is also a need to progress beyond health and disease models of ageing. Many valued aspects of human existence relate not only to health (Patrick 2003). Researchers also need to move away from 'professional centrism' (Stastny and Amering 1997) and ensure that their models and measurement instruments are grounded in lay perspectives (Ziller 1974; Fry 2000). The research reported here has also shown that adults of all ages within a society share a basic core of values, and older people are no different to younger people. But people in different social, cultural and demographic groups will inevitably emphasize and prioritize these differently. There is a need for measures of QoL to be more sensitive to this.

Each of the QoL themes mentioned here are also of potential relevance to frail people, and those who live in institutions and care homes (Beaumont and Kenealy 2004). They might also prioritize their privacy, ability to control their lives, the way they structure their days, a sense of self, features and quality of the environment, as well as their relationships, help and activities as most important (Clark and Bowling 1989, 1990; Qureshi et al. 1994; Fernàndez-Ballesteros 1998b; Tester et al. 2000; Weidekamp-Maicher 2001).

It should also be pointed out that many older people provide care for their spouses, especially when chronically and terminally ill (Schofield and Bloch 1998), and they themselves may simultaneously suffer from ill-health (Bowling and Cartwright 1982). Most people with chronic disability live at home, and some will require help with everyday and/or personal tasks. The provision of informal care can lead to considerable physical and emotional stress, and impact negatively on the carer's QoL (Hughes et al. 1999), although it can also lead to satisfaction and feelings of reciprocity (Murray et al. 1999). Few measures of QoL have been developed for this group, with the bulk of research being on specific domains determined by researchers' priorities and perspectives (e.g. stress). This is an area which requires a broader research focus.

In conclusion, more attention to differing values and priorities is needed in the conceptualization and measurement of QoL, as well as distinction between variables which influence, constitute and mediate QoL. And, given the diversity of measures used in QoL research, serious consideration needs to be given to the management of well calibrated pools of instruments. Such facilities are widely available for psychological tools, and attempts are now being made to introduce these for health-related QoL scales (Ware and Bayliss 2003).[1]

[1] This chapter is based, with permission, on a review of QoL by the author for the European Forum on Population Ageing Research (see Brown et al. 2004).

43

2

The study: aims, methods, measures, sample, response rates

Aims, methods and measures

This study set out to explore older people's definitions of, and priorities for, a good QoL. The questions it sought to address were:

- How do older people perceive and prioritize QoL?
- How do older people feel the quality of their lives can be improved?
- What are the main independent factors that influence QoL in older age?

Age 65 and over was taken to denote 'old age', which enabled comparisons to be made with other studies using this age cut-off point. As this was a survey of older age, rather than of growing older, people aged 65 and over were sampled rather than the over 50s, in order to provide the most information about this group. Old age is traditionally defined in relation to a specific birth anniversary, such as national state pension age. This traditional definition of old age is increasingly blurred as a result of early retirement and unemployment of older workers, and even by the very gradual introduction of flexible retirement age policy. It is, of course, acknowledged that any categorization by age is arbitrary and obscures the diversity of older people physiologically, psychologically and socially.

The research adopted a triangulated approach (using more than one method) within the same sample, in order to explore fully the respondents' perceptions of QoL. The survey respondents were interviewed using structured, semi-structured and in-depth interview methods. The survey questionnaire included open-ended questions, which elicited respondents' perceptions of a good and bad QoL, and how this could be improved, before standard scales, based on theoretically derived indicators of life quality, were administered. A sub-sample of respondents was followed up in greater depth using qualitative interview techniques, and all completed a postal follow-up questionnaire about 18 months later. Thus the research used both inductive and deductive methods of investigation and analysis.

The survey

Baseline measures

Open-ended QoL survey questions

A series of open-ended questions were asked at the beginning of the QoL survey interview in order to elicit respondents' descriptions of QoL, both good and bad, their priorities ('most important' area mentioned), how QoL can be improved for themselves and also for other people their age. Responses were recorded by hand by the interviewers (paper and pencil). These questions were followed by a self-rating of the quality of their lives overall on a seven-point Likert scale, derived from the SEIQoL response scales (using anchors from 'So good, it could not be better' to 'So bad, it could not be worse'; SPSS variable label 'MQL-9d') (Bowling, 1995a, 1995b; Hickey *et al.* 1999; Bowling *et al.* 2002a, 2003).

The open-ended questions were used as the opening survey questions in order to prevent respondent bias from the other, more specific, questions and scales included the questionnaire. They also built on existing open-ended questions on the important things in life (Bowling 1995a, 1995b, 1996). The open-ended survey questions on QoL are summarized below in Box 2.1 (and see Annex I for full versions).

Box 2.1 Open-ended survey questions

Thinking about your life as a whole, what is it that makes your life good – that is, the things that give your life quality? You may mention as many things as you like.

What is it that makes your life bad – that is the things that reduce the quality in your life? You may mention as many things as you like.

Thinking about all these good and bad things you have just mentioned, which one is the most important to you?

What single thing would improve the quality of your life?

What single thing, in your opinion, would improve the overall quality of life for people of your age?

The detailed coding frames for the open-ended survey responses were developed after AB and two coders read, independently, all of the interviewer scripts of responses, and were refined as coding took place over a six-week period. The coding was carried out by two coders and checked by AB. Main 'root' themes and detailed 'branch' sub-themes were coded in order to capture the essence of people's definitions and exactly what made their QoL good and bad, and how life could be improved (see Annex I in Chapters 4–9 for the broad theme 'roots' and the summaries of the detailed sub-theme 'branches'). These were all entered onto SPSS[10] as multi-coded items and merged with the main quantitative data set.

This categorization of open-ended survey responses represents a form of content analysis and should not be confused with qualitative research which employs smaller samples in order to provide deeper insights into people's lives, so as to understand their reasoning and perspectives. The analysis of open-ended survey responses is more limited, but nonetheless insightful in terms of providing the researcher with the wide range of understandings and interpretations of concepts that people use.

Structured survey measures

The hypothesis underlying the choice of structured survey measures, and their analysis, was that QoL is influenced by several factors, including social networks and support, health, psychological resources and characteristics, social capital, financial situation, independence, socioeconomic and sociodemographic characteristics. These themes, and their measurement, were derived from the literature. Thus, the open-ended questions on perceptions of QoL were followed by structured items and scales measuring these dimensions. In addition, the Office for National Statistics (ONS) Question Testing Unit organized three focus groups with older people to further inform the content of the questionnaire. The details of these structured items and scales are summarized next (and see Annex II for further details of items, and Annex III for further tests of reliability and validity).

Psychological resources

◆ Perceptions of self-efficacy (control and mastery over life; SPSS variable label 'EFFIC'), including self-ratings of perceived 'control over the important things in life' on three-point Likert scales from 'A lot, some, a little'; perceived ability to make successful plans, and action in the face of failure on five-point Likert scales from 'Strongly agree' to 'Strongly disagree' (Schwarzer 1993).

- Optimism-pessimism bias ('OPTIMIST') which included attitude statements about 'looking on the "bright side" ' and 'expect the best in uncertain times' on five-point Likert scales from 'Strongly agree' to 'Strongly disagree' (Sheier and Carver 1985).

- Real-unreal optimism-pessimism: perceived risks of negative life and negative health events ('RISKTOT'), including frailty and entering residential care ('RISKFRAI'), adverse health events, including frailty ('RISKHLTH'), accident or assault ('RISKASAC'). Respondents were asked to estimate their chances of listed events as 'Higher, about the same, or lower' in comparison with other men/women their age in Britain (men were asked to compare themselves with men, and women were asked to compare themselves with women) (Sutton 1998).

- Social comparisons and expectations, including self-ratings of living conditions, finances, achievements and health ('GAPTOTAL') in comparison with relevant others, or in comparison with their past circumstances and expectations, using five-point Likert scales from 'A lot worse off' to 'A lot better off', or three-point Likert scales 'More than expected, the same or less than expected'; and a five-point Likert scale measuring the extent of met achievements from 'I have done none of the things I wanted to' to 'I have done everything I wanted to'.

- Health values ('HEALVAL'), which included attitude statements on caring about other things 'more than one's health' and whether there were things 'more important than one's health', rated on five-point Likert scales from 'Strongly agree' to 'Strongly disagree' (Lau *et al.* 1986).

Physical health and functioning

- Functional status, including performance of activities and instrumental activities of daily living, known as ADL and IADL respectively ('ADLTOT') (Townsend 1979; Bond and Carstairs 1982; Martin *et al.* 1988), in which respondents were asked to rate their level of ability in performing listed daily tasks on a four-point Likert scale from 'No difficulty' to 'Unable to do alone'.

- The SF-36 item on health perceptions ('MQL-15a'): 'In general, compared with other people your age, would you say that your current health is . . . Excellent, very good, good, fair or poor?' (Ware *et al.* 1993).

- Self-reported long-standing illness, disability or infirmity (abbreviated as LSI) ('MQL-16a') ('yes/no' responses, with the positive responses followed up with questions on whether the condition affected their lives, and its duration).

◆ Plus self-reported, diagnosed medical conditions using a checklist of a range of conditions.

Psychological morbidity Psychological health was measured with the General Health Questionnaire, 12-item version (GHQ-12) which measures general non-psychotic psychiatric morbidity, including anxiety and depression ('GHQ-SCORE' and GHQCASE'). This uses four-point Likert scales rating feelings over the past week (e.g. from 'Better than usual' to 'Much less than usual') and also includes items on happiness and self-worth (Goldberg and Williams 1988)).

Social resources and social capital

a) Personal social resources, or personal social capital:

◆ Available help and support, if needed, with practical things in life, and total number of practical things can ask for help with ('PRACHELP'); personal support in a crisis ('COMFORT'); total number of practical and personal areas of life can ask for help with ('SUPTOT') (Sherbourne and Stewart 1991; Coulthard *et al.* 2001; Walker *et al.* 2001).

◆ Several questions covering numbers and type of helpers/supporters, frequency and type of social contacts and helpers; proximity of friends and relatives; summed frequency of contact with relatives and friends ('SOCTOT') (Sherbourne and Stewart 1991; Coulthard *et al.* 2001; Walker *et al.* 2001).

◆ Frequency and changes in loneliness ('MQL-14c and MQL-14g').

◆ Number and type of social activities ('ACTIVTOT'), as well as enjoyment of each.

b) External, or neighbourhood social capital:

◆ Enjoyment of living in the area and ratings of the quality of facilities in the area ('AREATOT') such as shops, transport, somewhere nice to go for a walk, on five-point Likert scales from 'Very good' to 'Very poor'.

◆ Rating of problems in the area ('PROBTOT'), including crime, litter, noise, pollution, graffiti, vandalism, on five-point Likert scales from 'A very big problem' to 'It doesn't happen'.

◆ Feelings of safety ('SAFETOT') (five-point scales from 'Very safe' to 'Very unsafe').

◆ Reported neighbourliness of area ('NEIGHBOR'): knowledge and trust of people in the neighbourhood, rated on a four-point scale ranging from 'Most people' to 'Do not know people in the neighbourhood' (Cooper *et al.* 1999; Coulthard *et al.* 2001; Walker *et al.* 2001).

Standard ONS Omnibus Survey items   Measures of sociodemographic and socioeconomic characteristics (both new and old standard classifications of socioeconomic status were used in order to facilitate comparisons between past and current studies), income, region of residence, a population density index encompassing number of population per hectare, and Acorn data (*A Classification of Residential Neighbourhoods*) were used to classify affluence of area of residence (see Annex II).

Mode of administering the interview schedule

The survey interview was based on computer-assisted interviewing with a laptop personal computer (PC). The interviewer showed the respondents how to key their responses into the PC in answer to each question. They then offered all respondents the choice of typing their own responses directly onto the PC themselves. Sixty-seven per cent accepted full or partial self-completion with the PC, and 32% preferred the interviewer to key in all their responses (1% did not reply). For 55% of respondents, this was their first time using the computer. Older respondents, aged 75+, were more likely to say this was the first time they had used a computer than those aged 65–74: 59% and 42% respectively. And 53% of women, compared to 47% of men, said this was the first time they had used a computer. National survey data for England show that 48% of men and 39% of women aged 65+ own a computer, although these figures declined with older age (Marmot *et al.* 2003). However, national statistics for Britain show that just 15% of people aged 65 and over had used the internet, although 44% of those aged 55–64 had done so (Office for National Statistics 2002). The figures from the QoL survey indicate that more would potentially use a computer if they had one in their homes. Whether they would use one to access the internet at home is more questionable, given current internet connection and broadband charges.

Survey follow-up

The follow-up questionnaire was a self-administered postal questionnaire, and thus needed to be concise. It was administered approximately 18 months after baseline home interview. The follow-up survey questionnaire duplicated the key baseline questions on self-rated QoL, difficulties with activities of daily living, long-standing illness and health status to enable changes in status between baseline and follow-up surveys to be calculated (change scores, and effect sizes). ADL score at follow-up was based on a subset of the baseline ADL, IADL and mobility items (walking 400 yards, getting on a bus, cutting toenails, going up/down steps/stairs, doing heavy housework, shopping and carrying heavy bags, bending to pick something up off the floor). Thus, the change variables were: change in ADL score ('ADLCHANG'); change in long-standing illness ('LSICHANG'); change in health status ('HEACHANG'); change in QoL rating ('QOLCHANG'). Scores were interpreted as 'deteriorated', 'unchanged' or 'improved'.

The opportunity was also taken to enquire about new topics. Open-ended questions (responses were categorized in the office) were asked about attitudes to ageing (see Box 2.2), and about major life changes in the last six months. Other items covered familial longevity, health behaviours, informal help and health service use.

Box 2.2 Attitudes to ageing – follow-up survey questions

What do you think are the best things about growing older? Please can you write what these are here? ('FMQL13a-f')

What do you think are the worst things about growing older? Please can you write what these are here? (FMQL14a-f')

What are your biggest fears about growing older? Please can you write what these are here? ('FMQL15a-f')

At what age do you consider someone to be old (precoded from 50<55 in five-year age bands up to 100 and over)? ('FMQL17')

Self-perceived age

Do you feel younger, older, or about the same as your actual age? (FMQL18a)

If you feel younger or older: about what age do you feel you are? ('FMQL18b')

Please write in the age you feel – – – years.

A computed variable was created from the two self-perceived age items combining whether the respondents felt older, younger or the same as their actual age, with the actual number of years they felt older or younger than their own age ('DIFFFEEL').

Statistics

Statistics used for survey analyses

Statistical tests were used to give some indication of the probability of differences occurring by chance, and they informed the decision about which results to present. The results of statistical testing are not always given in the text, partly to facilitate its readability, and partly because of the spurious precision they can imply (so caution in interpretation is needed, given the large number of tests that were carried out, as some results will inevitably be due to chance). Unless otherwise stated, attention is not drawn to differences which statistical testing indicates might have occurred by chance 5 or more times in 100.

Not all cross-analyses of the data which were conducted are presented here, although standard analyses with sociodemographic and socioeconomic variables were carried out with the main variables presented in each chapter. While positive associations are reported, not all negative or inconclusive associations are reported, again for reasons of simplicity of presentation.

The variables of interest from the survey data were explored using univariate analyses (frequency distributions), and bivariate analyses (chi-square tests and zero-order correlations). Wilcoxon signed rank test was used to compare differences over time (baseline and follow-up surveys). As the data were weighted, the sub-totals and totals of the frequencies and cross-tabulations are not always consistent in the dataset but may vary by a small number (see p. 52).

Hierarchical multiple regression was used to analyse the independent effects of theoretically relevant and statistically significant independent variables on the dependent variables of interest (self-rated QoL; changes in QoL; subjective age or age-identity). Hierarchical regression was selected as it is theory driven not data driven, and enables theory-relevant hypotheses to be tested (Sciafa and Games 1987). The variables which were entered into regression models were those of theoretical relevance, and most, although not all, had achieved statistical significance, using chi-square tests and zero-order correlations (Spearman's rank order correlations) at the bivariate level. Demographic and socioeconomic variables were included into models last, regardless of prior statistical significance, as they were considered as *a priori* hypotheses on the basis of a broad range of literature. The independent variables entered into the regression model of self-rated QoL were entered in themed clusters, and were also represented in the broader lay models of QoL, with the exception of self-assessed risks of adverse life events.

Multi-colinearity was assessed beforehand for each of the models, firstly by examining the zero-order correlations between the subjective ranked variables (Spearman's rank order correlation was used). These satisfied the 0.7 bivariate threshold for entry (Tabachnick and Fidell 2001). As these correlations were limited to bivariate analyses, multi-colinearity was assessed secondly by examining the tolerance values for the variables entered into the regression analysis (colinearity diagnostics within the SPSS regression analysis). These were all high (between 0.7 and 0.9) indicating that multi-colinearity was at a respectable level (low values near 0 indicate multiple correlation with other entered variables), and thereby justifying the entry of the variables (Katz 1999).

Survey sample

The QoL survey aimed to identify all respondents aged 65+, living at home, to four quarterly ONS Omnibus Surveys in Britain, and to include them in the QoL survey. This enabled seasonal effects to be controlled for and recruitment of a sample size large enough to generate a wide range of items about QoL, to permit cross-tabulations with the variables proposed. All respondents aged 65 and over who were interviewed for the Omnibus Survey (April, September, November 2000; January 2001) were asked at the end of that interview if they would be willing to be re-interviewed by ONS interviewers for our module on QoL. Those who consented to participate further were re-interviewed for the QoL survey two months after their Omnibus Survey interview.

The sampling frame used for the Omnibus Survey was the British postcode address file of 'small users'. This file includes all private household addresses. Postal sectors were stratified by region, the proportion of households renting from local authorities, and the proportion in which the head of household is in socioeconomic group 1–5 or 13 (i.e. a professional, employer or manager). A hundred postal sectors were selected with probability proportional to size. Within each sector, 30 addresses were selected randomly with a target sample size per survey of about 2000 adults aged 16 and over (one per sampled household with the use of a random numbers table). Because only one household member is interviewed, people in households containing few adults had a better chance of selection than those in households with many. A weighting factor was applied to correct for this unequal probability.

Response and profile of survey respondents

The overall (combined) response rate for the four main Omnibus Surveys from which our QoL survey members were sifted (April, June, September,

Table 2.1 Response rates to Omnibus Survey and QoL survey

	(n)	%	
Omnibus (sift) survey response			
Selected addresses	12,000	100	
Ineligible addresses	1,089	9	
Eligible addresses	10,909		
Refusals	3,034	28	
Non-contacts	1,164	11	
Interviews achieved	6,711	62	
Omnibus survey interviews achieved with people aged 65+	1,598	100	
Agreement to re-interview for QoL survey	1,323	83	
Refused re-interview for QoL survey	275	17	
QoL survey response			
Selected individuals	1,323	100	
Ineligible individuals	24	2	
Eligible individuals	1,299		
Refusals on re-contact	243	19	
Non-contacts during QoL fieldwork stage	57	4	
Interviews achieved +	999	77 (or, 63% of the 1598 Omnibus Survey respondents aged 65+)	
(+ includes seven partial interviews)			

Note: There were a total of 1598 respondents to the April, June, September and November Omnibus Surveys aged 65 years and over. Of these, 275 (17%) refused any further contact by interviewers, and so were not included as part of the QoL sample above.
Source: Bowling *et al.* (2002a)

November 2000) was 62% (6711) (range over the four surveys: 57–65%); this is shown above in Table 2.1 (and see Bowling *et al.* 2002a). ONS sifted 1299 eligible respondents from these surveys who were eligible for inclusion in the QoL survey. The overall response rate for the QoL survey was 77% (999) (range over the four waves: 69–83%); 19% refused to participate and 4% were not contactable during the interview period.

Thus, 999 randomly-sampled people aged 65 and over, living at home in Britain, were interviewed for the QoL survey. The interviews took place in respondents' own homes in July, September, November and December 2000 and February 2001. The interviews lasted between 60 and 90 minutes. While lengthy, respondents and interviewers commented that they enjoyed the broad-ranging interview.

The sociodemographic characteristics of all adult respondents (aged 16+) to the *initial four ONS Omnibus Surveys* (for the sifting of eligible QoL survey respondents) were very similar to those of respondents to the ONS General Household Survey (GHS) and similar to mid-year population estimates for Great Britain (estimated from the last census) in relation to most variables compared (e.g. for gender, ethnicity, housing tenure). The exception was with younger respondents – the ONS Omnibus Survey under-represented people aged under 44. The percentage of Omnibus respondents aged 65 and over was very similar to that expected from their distribution in the population (this was the group eligible for the QoL survey, where they consented). In total, 24% of all adult respondents to the full Omnibus Survey were aged 65+.

The *respondents to the subsequent QoL survey* were similar in their sociodemographic characteristics to those of people aged 65+ in Britain from mid-term population estimates from the 1991 Census, and compared with respondents aged 65+, living at home, in the comparable GHS and other national surveys (Bridgwood 2000; Walker *et al.* 2001; Falaschetti *et al.* 2002). The only difference was that the QoL sample had slightly fewer women (48%) than might be expected (58% of people in the general population aged 65+ are women). A small amount of selection bias may have operated, apart from excluding people (who are mainly women) who live in residential care and nursing homes – for example, it is possible that iller and more busy women were among the non-responders.

More detailed comparisons by age group can also be made with respondents to the module for people aged 65+ in the 1998 GHS (Bridgwood 2000). (The published 2000 GHS presents fewer detailed age group comparisons among people aged 65 and over.) Again, the QoL survey respondents were broadly similar in the distributions of their characteristics. For example, 33% (330) lived alone, a figure identical to the 1998 GHS respondents. In addition, 69% (692) of QoL survey members owned their own home outright, 7% (68) owned their home on a mortgage and 24% (238) rented their home (the 1998 distributions were similar with, for example, two-thirds being owner-occupiers). 62% (615) of QoL respondents reported a long-standing illness (LSI), disability or infirmity, in comparison with 61% to the 1998 GHS. The surveys compared well, with most reported LSIs attributed to musculoskeletal disorders and heart and circulatory conditions, with no differences between cause and sex of respondents except with musculoskeletal conditions (more women reported these). Further, 70% of respondents aged 65+ reported an LSI to the Health Survey for England in 2000 (Falaschetti *et al.* 2002), but thissample included people living in residential care and nursing homes, thus a higher figure would be expected.

Follow-up response rates

Out of the 999 baseline survey respondents, 786 (79%) had agreed to be recontacted, and 533 of these (68%) returned the completed postal questionnaire about 18 months later. There were no differences in sociodemographic or health characteristics between the responders and the non-responders to baseline or follow-up studies, or between the baseline consenters and non-consenters to follow-up. They were also broadly representative of people aged 65 and over living at home in Britain (Bridgwood *et al.* 2000).

The strength of the study design was that the baseline sample was a national random sample of people aged 65+, who were interviewed at home, a high proportion of whom consented to be followed up and returned their follow-up postal questionnaires. Of course, this left a substantial minority who did not respond, although analysis of the characteristics of responders and non-responders revealed no major differences between groups. A potential weakness of the study was that the sample did not include people living in institutions, or those with any evidence of mental confusion, as interviewers were instructed to terminate such interviews on the grounds of validity of reported information. Thus the results presented here relate to mentally able people aged 65 and over living in their own homes. Caution in the generalization of the results is needed, as the responders to the study may also be an elite – the 'successful survivors'.

Characteristics of QoL survey respondents

So who were the people in the QoL sample? The baseline sample was evenly divided between men and women, and most (just under two-thirds) were aged 65<74. Most were married although over a quarter were widowed and a third lived alone. The vast majority of respondents were white, as would be expected in a national sample of people aged 65 and over. Tables 2.2a to 2.2c show the detailed characteristics of respondents at baseline.

Table 2.2b also shows respondents' educational level, access to resources and details of socioeconomic status and area of residence. There were few

Table 2.2a Sociodemographic characteristics of survey respondents

	%
Sex	
Male	52
Female	48
Age	
65–74	62
75+	38
Marital status	
Single, never married	5
Married/cohabiting	62
Married, separated from spouse	1
Divorced	5
Widowed	27
Ethnic status	
White	98
Black Caribbean	1
Other	1
No. of respondents	**998–999**

Table 2.2b Socioeconomic status characteristics of survey respondents

	%
Age left full-time education	
Up to 14+	48
15–18	41
19–25	8
Over 25	3
(+ includes five who did not receive any education)	
Highest education qualification	
Degree or higher degree	6
Higher educational qualification below degree	6
A levels or higher	4
ONC/BTEC	2

O level or GSCE equivalent	8
GCSE grade D–E or GCSE grade 2–5	1
Other	9
No formal qualifications	64

Gross annual income before tax

Less than £4,160	23
£4,160 < £6,240	24
£6,240 < £9,360	22
£9,360 < £17,680	21
£17,680 or more	10

In paid work in last 7 days

Yes	5
No	95

Socioeconomic group (if ever had paid job)

Professional	5
Employers and managers	19
Intermediate non-manual	14
Junior non-manual	15
Skilled manual	23
Semi-skilled manual	18
Unskilled	6

Social class (old coding)

I Professional	5
II Intermediate	28
III Non-manual, skilled non manual	20
III Manual, skilled manual	24
IV Partly skilled	16
V Unskilled	7
VI Armed forces	–

Social class (new coding) (n=972)

Employers and managers, large organizations	9
Higher professionals	19
Lower managerial, professional	15

(Continued)

Table 2.2b Continued

	%
Intermediate occupations	13
Small employers, own account workers	7
Lower supervisory, crafts etc.	13
Semi-routine occupations	23
Routine occupations	10
Car/van available to household	
Yes	67
No	33
No. of respondents	**972–999**

Table 2.2c Area and household characteristics of survey respondents

	%
Region of residence	
North	25
Midlands and East Anglia	28
London	7
South East	14
South West	13
Wales	5
Scotland	8
Acorn categorization: affluence of respondent's area of residence	
Thriving	26
Expanding	8
Rising	6
Settling	29
Aspiring	16
Striving	15
Number of adults in household	
1	33
2	60
3	7

Type of household	
One person only	33
Married/cohabiting – no dependent children	59
Lone parent – no dependent children	1
Other	7
Respondent's own housing tenure	
Owns home outright	69
Owns home on mortgage/loan	7
Rents	24
Lives here rent free	–
No. of respondents	**968 – 999**

Tables 2.2a–c: Due to sample weighting totals do not always equal 100%.

opportunities for higher education for the majority of respondents when they were young. As would be expected in this age group, almost half had left school at age 14 or below and almost two-thirds had no formal qualifications. Just tiny percentages had a degree or higher degree.

Their lack of qualifications had repercussions for both their occupations and incomes when working, and their pensions in retirement. Almost half the sample fell into the lower socioeconomic classes, and almost half received an annual income of less than £6240 (e.g. those without occupational pensions, and who thus relied on their state pensions). Just a tiny percentage was still in paid work. Of course, lowered incomes in retirement are partly offset by the expectation that home owners have paid off their mortgages, and this was the case for most; but this still left almost a third who were either renting their homes or still paying off their mortgages.

Another commonly used indicator of social deprivation is access to a car or van within the household. While most had such access, a large percentage (a third) of respondents had no access to a car or van (e.g. due to poor health, low incomes or loss of a spouse who was relied on for driving). As will be illustrated in Chapter 9, access to transport was often vital for retaining social participation and independence. Many people commented that they had no access to good public transport, or they did not feel safe using public transport at night, and were thus effectively isolated (see Chapter 7). This is perhaps unsurprising given that over a third of people lived in the two lowest density population

---

Box 2.3 Acorn area prosperity categories

A 'Thriving' (1 wealthy achievers, suburban areas, 2 affluent greys, rural communities, 3 prosperous pensioners, retirement areas).

B 'Expanding' (4 affluent executives, family areas, 5 well-off workers, family areas).

C 'Rising' (6 affluent urbanites, town and city areas, 7 prosperous professionals, metropolitan areas, 8 better-off executives, inner city areas).

D 'Settling' (9 comfortable middle-agers, mature home owning areas, 10 skilled workers, home owning areas).

E 'Aspiring' (11 new home owners, mature communities, 12 white-collar workers, better-off multi-ethnic areas).

F 'Striving' (13 older people, less prosperous areas, 14 council estate residents, better-off homes, 15 council estate residents, high unemployment, 16 council estate residents, greatest hardship, 17 people in multi-ethnic, low-income areas).

---

bands (indicating rural, remote neighbourhoods) and about a quarter lived in the two highest population bands (e.g. inner-city, densely populated areas); many of the latter can be classified as 'striving' (least affluent – see Box 2.3 for more detailed Acorn definitions). For example, just 4% of people who lived in the most affluent, 'thriving', Acorn areas were also within the highest population density band (3824–11,931), far more, 17%, of those living in the least affluent, 'striving', areas fell into this highest population density band.

In-depth follow-up interviews

With the aim of obtaining a better understanding of people's interpretations of QoL, in-depth interviews about QoL were carried out about 18 months later with a sub-sample of 80 of the 999 participants in the QoL survey. These in-depth interviews were also repeated one year on.

In-depth interview approach

The subsequent in-depth interviews with a sub-sample of respondents were based on semi-biographical interview techniques, with QoL in older age viewed as a developmental process, rather than a stage of life, with perceptions of QoL coloured by past, as well as present, experiences and circumstances. The assumption behind this approach was that the meaning of QoL in older age cannot be separated from the rest of the life course. The interviews followed the grounded theory approach of enabling themes to emerge from respondents' own stories.

The interview technique aimed to enable themes to emerge from respondents' own stories, to facilitate people talking about QoL in the context of their overall lives, and to enhance the researchers' understanding of people's perspectives on life. Respondents were first asked to describe key events in their lives, including marriage, work and/or parenthood where relevant. Then the interviewer used a checklist and asked respondents what they thought of when they heard the words 'quality of life', to describe their QoL, what gave their lives quality and what took quality away from their lives, how it could be improved, what would make it worse and about any changes since the survey interview. The interviews were conducted by Zahava Gabriel (ZG). They lasted approximately 60 minutes, and were audio-recorded and transcribed.

The detailed coding frames for the in-depth interviews were developed after ZG and AB read all of the scripts of responses, and were refined as coding took place. Where there was overlap, the categories used for the open-ended survey interviews were used to facilitate comparisons. The thematic coding was carried out by ZG and checked independently by AB.

Brief telephone interviews were conducted with each in-depth interview respondent exactly one year after their in-depth interview had taken place. These interviews elicited changes in the lives of half of the respondents, and these people were then re-interviewed face-to-face in order to explore these further.

The in-depth interview sample members and their characteristics

The intention was to interview a broad cross-section of respondents to the QoL survey. Thus seven quota matrices were designed with the aim of obtaining a sociodemographically varied sample, including variations in respondents' baseline sociodemographic characteristics, income, health and functional status, QoL ratings and region of residence. Participants were then purposively sampled by applying the matrices to the sample of 999 respondents. In order to achieve the target of 80 in-depth interviews, 106 respondents were approached and 80 were successfully interviewed (10 of the 106 had moved and 16 refused).

The in-depth follow-up sample purposively included 40 men and 40 women, ranging in age from 65 to over 80 (26 were aged 65<70, 20 were 70<75, 20 were 75<80 and 14 were 80+); 37 were married and the rest were single, never married (5), married but separated (1), divorced (6) or widowed (31); 36 had an income of less than £6240 per annum, and the rest had more than this. Twenty-five of the 80 respondents were categorized as having an excellent or good functional ability (performance at everyday tasks and mobility), 43 as fair, and the remainder as poor. Thirty-five rated their overall QoL as 'So good, it could not be better' or as 'Very good', 28 rated it as 'Good', ten rated it as 'Alright' and the remainder said it was 'Bad'/'Very bad' or 'So bad, it could not be worse'. They represented six widely spread geographical regions of England and Scotland.

Annex I: open-ended QoL questions

We are interested in finding out about what makes your life good and bad – that is, your quality of life – and the things that increase and reduce the quality of your life.

For most of this interview I will be recording your answers to questions on the computer. Just for the first two questions, I will be asking you to tell me about things in your own words and I will be writing your answers down on paper as you tell me.

First of all, thinking about your life as a whole, what is it that makes your life good – that is, the things that give your life quality? You may mention as many things as you like.

(*INTERVIEWER PROBE*: What is it about this that makes your life good? *INTERVIEWER RECORD VERBATIM*)

And what is it that makes your life bad – that is the things that reduce the quality in your life? You may mention as many things as you like.

(*INTERVIEWER PROBE*: What is it about this that reduces it? *INTERVIEWER RECORD VERBATIM*)

REFER TO PAPER – RECORD ON COMPUTER

Thinking about all these good and bad things you have just mentioned, which one is the most important to you?

Again, thinking about the good and bad things you have mentioned that make up your quality of life, which of the answers on this card best describes the quality of your life as a whole?

(1) So good, it could not be better
(2) Very good
(3) Good
(4) Alright

(5) Bad

(6) Very bad

(7) So bad, it could not be worse

And what single thing would improve the quality of your life?

And what single thing, in your opinion, would improve the overall quality of life for people of your age?

Annex II: measures used in the QoL survey
(Bowling and Gabriel 2004)

- Perceptions of self-efficacy (mastery and control: 'How much control do you feel you have over the important things in your life?', with three-point Likert response statements: 'A lot of control', 'Some control', 'Little/no control'; 'Things never work out the way I want them to'; 'When I make plans I am certain to make them work'; 'Failure just makes me try harder', each with five-point Likert scales from 'Strongly disagree' to 'Strongly agree') (Schwarzer 1993). (SPSS computed (scored) variable name: 'EFFIC'. For a small number of exploratory analyses a total score was also computed combining scores on optimism, self-efficacy and health values: SPSS variable name 'EFFICACY'.)
- Optimism-pessimism bias ('In uncertain times I usually expect the best'; 'I always look on the bright side of things', with five-point Likert scales from 'Strongly disagree' to 'Strongly agree') (Scheier and Carver 1985). (SPSS computed (scored) variable name: 'OPTIMIST'.)
- Real-unreal optimism-pessimism: perceived risks of life events in comparison with other men/women of the same age (being mugged, being burgled, falling and breaking a bone, being knocked down when crossing the road, suffering from selected (where unreported) medical conditions: cancer, heart disease, losing memory, becoming housebound, entering a nursing home). An additional item on living to be a 100 years old was added at the end (Sutton 1998). (SPSS computed (scored) variable name with both life and health events ('RISKTOT'), frailty-related risk events only (becoming housebound, admission to nursing home) ('RISKFRAI'), and risk events with health events (including frailty) only ('RISKHLTH'), risk of accident or assault only ('RISKASAC').)
- Social comparisons and expectations for financial and living circumstances, life aspirations and achievements: 'I would like you to think about your current living conditions and financial situation. Compared with what you had when you were in your 40s, which of these statements best applies to you?' and 'Compared to those around you (those like yourself, and who you compare yourself with), which statement best applies to you?' – both with five-point Likert scale statements, 'I am a lot worse off' to 'I am a lot better off'. 'Thinking about the things you have done in your

life and the things you would like to have done, which statement on the card best applies to you?' with five-point Likert scale statements, 'I have done none of the things I wanted to do' to 'I have done everything I wanted to do'. Expectations: 'And compared with what you expected you would have at this time in your life when you were in your 40s, would you say you had . . .', with three-point Likert scale statements, 'More than expected' to 'Less than expected') ('GAP').

◆ Health expectations and comparisons: 'Compared with how you expected your health to be at this time in your life, is your current health better, the same, or worse than you expected?' ('MQL-15b'). 'In general, compared with other people your age, would you say that your current health is excellent, very good, good, fair or poor?' (MQL-15a, SF-36 Health Perceptions item) ('GAPHEALT') (additive score of financial and living, aspirations and health expectations and comparisons: 'GAPTOTAL').

◆ Health values: 'There are many things I care about more than my health'; 'There are few things more important than good health', with five-point Likert scales from 'Strongly disagree' to 'Strongly agree') (Lau *et al.* 1986). (SPSS computed (scored) variable name: 'HEALTVAL'.)

◆ Level of functional ability in self-care, home-care and mobility were measured using the Townsend ADL scale (Townsend 1979; Bond and Carstairs 1982) and also supplemented with items on physical and sensory functioning from the ONS Disability Scale (Martin *et al.* 1988). (SPSS computed (scored) variable name of Townsend items: 'ADLTOT'.) Items included: walk at least 100 yards, put one arm behind back (dressing), tie a bow in shoelaces, get in/out of chair, count well enough to manage money, eat, drink and digest food, get on a bus, wash self all over, cut toenails, go up/down steps/stairs, heavy housework, shopping and carrying heavy bags, prepare and cook a hot meal, reaching for something on overhead shelf, bend down to pick something off the floor, balance when standing, control bladder, see well enough to read a newspaper, hear a conversation against background noise, understand what people say or mean, get up and do things (energy).

◆ Perceived health status, compared with others of same age: SF-36 item on health perceptions ('MQL-15a') (Ware *et al.* 1993).

◆ Reported long-standing illness, disability or infirmity, using the standard ONS question (MQL-16a), and restriction on activities.

◆ Medical conditions: falls and diagnosed medical conditions (heart, stroke and circulatory conditions, high blood pressure, asthma, chronic bronchitis, depression, panic attacks, agoraphobia, cancer, osteoporosis, rheumatoid arthritis, osteoarthritis, gout, other arthritis).

◆ Psychological morbidity (GHQ-12 which detects mainly anxiety and depression, and which also includes single items on ability to concentrate, worry, self-esteem (playing a useful part in things; confidence in self; feelings of worthlessness), decision-making, strain, ability to overcome difficulties, enjoyment, facing up to problems, happiness, unhappiness). (SPSS computed (scored) variable name and computed cases: 'GHQSCORE', 'GHQCASE' – Goldberg and Williams 1988.)

♦ Receipt of social and health services.
♦ Personal social capital (perceived social network structure and support) (Sherbourne and Stewart 1991; Coulthard *et al.* 2001; Walker *et al.* 2001) (SPSS computed (scored) variable names):
  ♦ Frequency score for contacts with relatives and friends ('SOCTOT').
  ♦ Frequency of social contact by phone, face to face and/or email with sons and daughters, brothers and sisters, other relatives, friends, neighbours, time proximity and geographical spread (MQL-46a-50).
  ♦ Number of practical/instrumental areas can ask for help with, type of helper, time proximity of residences proximity (lift, help if ill, borrow money, everyday chores (errands, odd jobs) ('PRACHELP')).
  ♦ Has someone to turn to for comfort/support in serious personal crisis ('COMFORT').
  ♦ Number of areas of life in total can ask for help with – emotional plus practical areas ('SUPTOT').
♦ Frequency of, and changes in, loneliness ('MQL-14c' and 'MQL-14g' respectively).
♦ Number of activities – clubs, local organizations, groups, evening/educational class, place of worship, cinema, theatre, place of entertainment, voluntary work, game or sport, swimming, keep fit, dancing, walking, library, gardening, child-minding, carer of someone ill/frail, other ('ACTIVTOT'); voting ('MQL-43'); importance of activities; frequency of getting out of house ('MQL-44'), holidays/outings ('MQL-45').
♦ External social capital: perceptions of the local area 'within about a 15–20 minute walk/drive from home' (e.g. ratings of itemized facilities, neighbourliness, safety, problems); social and civic engagement (community involvement, voting, feeling able to influence events within the community); reciprocity and local trust (number of local people knows and trusts) (Cooper *et al.* 1999; Walker *et al.* 2001). These were measured as follows:
  ♦ Enjoyment of living in area; ratings of availability of social and leisure activities ('for people like yourself'); facilities for people aged 65+; rubbish collection; local health services; local transport; closeness to shops; somewhere nice to walk ('AREATOT').
  ♦ Problems within the area (noise, crime, air quality, litter, graffiti) ('PROBTOT').
  ♦ Safety of the area (feels safe walking alone in area during day, after dark) ('SAFETOT').
  ♦ Control over area (feels can influence decisions that affect area) ('MQL-36').
  ♦ Reported neighbourliness of area ('NEIGHBOR') (i) knows (ii) trusts many/ most/few/none of people in neighbourhood.
♦ Standard ONS Omnibus Survey sociodemographic and socioeconomic characteristics and classifications (both old and new classifications of social class were used).

♦ Standard ONS Omnibus Survey classifications of population density (number of population per hectare) and Acorn classifications of area affluence (see Box 2.3, p. 60). Acorn (A Classification of Residential Neighbourhoods) classifications consist of six categories (17 groups and 54 types) and were developed from items in the 1991 census, at enumeration district level, including age, marital status, household size, housing tenure, car ownership, unemployment, occupation, ethnic status and reported long-term illness. Using postcodes, survey respondents were classified according to the Acorn categorization of the enumeration districts in which they lived. The six Acorn categories can be ranked along a dimension representing level of prosperity (see Box 2.3, p. 60).

Annex III: reliability and validity of the structured measures used

Reliability

The reliability of the scaled domains included in the questionnaire was assessed using tests of internal consistency. For example, the internal consistency reliability of the scaled and scored measures used was supported by their Cronbach's alpha statistics: GHQ-12 (alpha: 0.83); physical functioning (Townsend ADL scale) (0.91); perception of risk of adverse events sub-sections and overall (0.59–0.74); self-efficacy sub-sections and overall scale (0.34–0.41); control over life sub-scale (0.41); optimism-pessimism (0.51); social comparisons and expectations – financial (0.61); social comparisons and expectations – financial plus health (0.58); quality of (0.64) and problems in area of residence (0.65); neighbourliness of area (0.64); social support (0.60); practical help (0.61).

Validity

Where scales and computed variables tapped similar or overlapping concepts, there were moderate and significant correlations between them ranging from 0.05 to 0.001 levels of confidence, supporting their validity.

The validity of the QoL self-rating uniscale was supported in correlation analyses. These showed that the uniscale was significantly, if modestly, correlated with theoretically relevant or related variables relating to specific constructs, in the expected directions (minus signs in front of correlation values reflects direction of coding/scoring). The strongest correlation with self-rated quality of life was with health status, which is supported by the literature (Bowling 1995b). For example, QoL was correlated with physical functioning (ADL score) (r: 0.30, $p<0.001$); perceived health status (r: 0.39, $p<0.001$); as well as with social comparisons and expectations (r: –0.27; $p<0.001$); self-efficacy (r: 0.23, $p<0.001$); optimism-pessimism (r: 0.10, $p<0.01$); depression/anxiety

(GHQ-12) (r: 0.31, p<0.001); number of social activities (r: –0.23, p<0.001); perceived social support (r: –0.19, p<0.001); and perceived quality of the area of residence (r: 0.22, p<0.001).

Other measures used in the survey questionnaire, which were theoretically expected to be associated with each other, were also significantly correlated (low to moderate) in the expected directions. For example, frequency of, and increase in, loneliness were correlated (r: 0.44, p<0.001); self-efficacy and depression/anxiety (r: 0.27, p<0.001); physical functioning (Townsend ADL score) and perceived health status (r: 0.49, p<0.001); social support and social activities (r: 0.22, p<0.001); social support and social contacts (r: –0.19, p<0.001). These correlations provide support for the construct validity of the measures used.

Items used to measure constructs of interest also had convergent validity. For example, in the self-rating of risk of adverse events scale, respondents who rated their chances of falling as higher than other men/women of the same age, were more likely to report that they had fallen in the last year (45%), than those who rated their chances as about the same (29% of these reported that they had fallen) or lower (17% of these reported that they had fallen).

The prevalence of LSI disability or infirmity (62%, 95% CI: 59–65) and any limitation on activities due to longstanding illness (LLSI) (40%, CI: 38–43) were similar to the levels reported in the successive GHS between 1995 and 1998 (Bridgwood *et al.* 2000). LSI and/or LLSI were strongly associated with self-reported diagnosed medical conditions (circulatory diseases, respiratory diseases, mental health problems and musculoskeletal diseases), corroborating earlier research (Schroll 1994; Ebrahim *et al.* 2000; Ayis *et al.* 2003). The percentage of respondents who reported an LSI was 17% (confidence interval: 15–19) among those with no reported diagnosed conditions, increasing to 91% (confidence interval 90–3) among those with five or more conditions (Ayis *et al.* 2003). This supports the construct validity of the item. The LSI question does reflect several well-documented biases. For example, people with chronic illnesses or disability do not always report they have a LSI, and older people may regard limitations in their daily activities, particularly those due to poor eyesight and hearing, as a normal part of ageing, rather than evidence of illness or disability (Goddard 1990 cited by Bridgwood 2000). Moreover, increases in the proportions of people reporting an LSI over time in successive waves of the GHS have been noted by ONS, with explanations ranging from increasing expectations to the increase in the numbers of people with chronic conditions (perhaps due to more successful, life-saving treatments) (Walker *et al.* 2001).

Estimates of ill-health among older people are, of course, underestimates in the survey presented here, as the sample did not include the 7% of older people living in communal establishments (hospitals, nursing homes, residential homes).

3

What adds quality to life, and what takes it away?

> Sooner or later in life, everyone discovers that perfect happiness is unrealisable, but there are few who pause to consider the antithesis: that perfect unhappiness is equally unattainable.
>
> Primo Levi (1958), *If this is a Man*, p. 23. Published by Jonathan Cape.
> Reprinted by permission of the Random House Group Ltd.

This chapter will present respondents' ratings and perceptions of QoL. It also compares the results of a multiple regression model of theoretically derived predictors of self-rated QoL with i) respondents' own perceptions of QoL (categorization of open-ended survey questions), and ii) with the views of a sub-sample who were followed up in greater depth. The open-ended responses and in-depth interviews were also of value as they provided context and meaning for the analysis of the composition of QoL, as well as broadening the development of a conceptual model of QoL in older age.

Theoretical model of QoL

Overall QoL ratings

The first research questions were: how do older people perceive and prioritize their QoL, and how do they feel it can be improved? After being asked for their views about QoL (see p. 45), respondents were asked to rate their overall QoL on a seven-point Likert scale, from 'So good, could not be better' to 'So bad, could not be worse'. There were no consistent seasonal effects with QoL ratings. Most men and women rated their QoL as good: 5% rated their QoL as 'So good it could not be better'; 77% said it was 'Very good' or 'Good'; 15% rated it as 'Alright'; only 3% said it was 'Bad' or 'Very bad'; and less than 1% rated it as 'So bad it could not be worse' (see Figure 3.1). It is commonly reported in textbooks on questionnaire methods that few people are inclined to rate

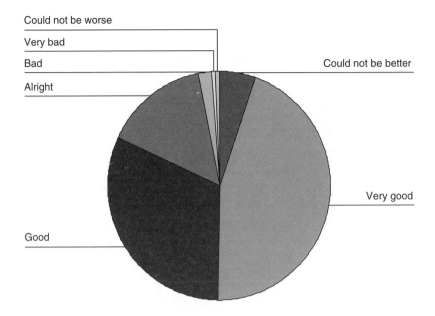

Figure 3.1 QoL ratings

themselves at the extremes (Bowling 2005). There were few differences with gender (see Figure 3.2).

However, as Figure 3.3 illustrates, QoL deteriorated with older age, with both men and women aged 65–69 reporting higher QoL ratings than older respondents: 71% of this youngest group rated their QoL as 'So good it could not be better' or 'Very good' in comparison with fewer, 51%, of those aged 70–74, 46% of those aged 75–79 and 32% of those aged 80+. This might be expected given that challenges in life often accumulate with age (e.g. bereavement, declining health and functioning).

Self-rated QoL was analysed in further detail. The research question guiding these analyses was: to what extent are self-evaluations of global QoL influenced, independently, by indicators of social, psychological and physical health, social capital, sociodemographic and socioeconomic status? The associations with self-rated QoL will be reported in the chapters that follow, and are summarized here (see also Bowling *et al.* 2002a for detailed breakdowns and tables).

Bivariate analyses showed that, in general, respondents who were in the highest socioeconomic groups, and with the most positive psychological outlooks, were more likely than others to rate their lives as 'So good it could

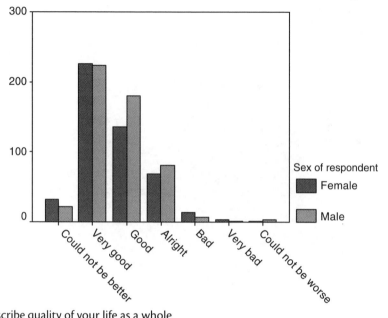

Describe quality of your life as a whole

Figure 3.2 QoL ratings by gender

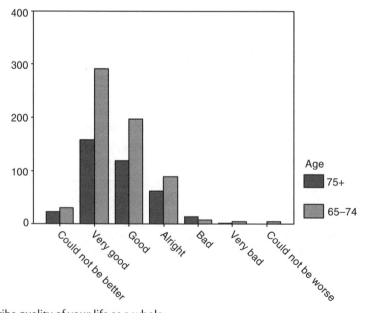

Describe quality of your life as a whole

Figure 3.3 QoL ratings by age

not be better' or 'Very good'. Thus they were more likely to have high self-efficacy; to make downward social comparisons and rate their financial and living situations as better than expected, and better compared with others ('gap' theory); they had no psychological morbidity; were optimistic in their outlooks, and rated themselves (optimistically) as at low risk of negative life and health events.

Those with the highest levels of personal social resources were also more likely than others to rate their QoL as 'Very good'. These respondents were more likely to have the greatest number of areas they could ask for help and support with; the highest number of social activities; they were not lonely; they were pet owners; and they had someone to turn to for comfort. They were also more likely to have the best neighbourhood social capital. For example, they were more likely to rate the quality of their area facilities and services as 'Very good', to report the least problems with crime, antisocial behaviour and so on in the neighbourhood; and to rate their areas as neighbourly and safe.

Those respondents with the best physical functioning, with no restrictions due to long-standing illness, with the best perceived health status, and in better health than they had expected to be, were more likely to rate their QoL as 'Very good'. The results for marital status were also statistically significant but more mixed, with those who were married, divorced or separated being more likely than those who were widowed or single to rate their lives as 'Very good'.

Regression analyses of the independent predictors of QoL ratings

In order to assess the relative contribution of the theoretically relevant variables to QoL self-ratings (dependent variable), a hierarchical multiple linear regression analysis was carried out on the 999 survey respondents (see Bowling *et al.* 2002a for detailed analyses), using the structured questionnaire data. The independent, predictor variables which were entered (in blocks where more than one per domain) were those which were measured using standardized scales and items:

1 Social comparisons and expectations computed gap scores (Model 1).

2 Personality and psychological variables computed scores (self-efficacy, optimism-pessimism bias, anxiety/depression, self-assessed risks of negative life events – accidents, assault) (Model 2).

3 Health and functional status items and computed scores (activities of daily living score, self-assessed health status, reported long-standing illness) (Model 3).

4 Social capital (personal) computed variables (number of social activities, frequency of social contacts score, amount of help and social support, pet owner, frequency of loneliness, increase in loneliness) (Model 4).

5 Social capital (local neighbourhood) computed variables (quality rating of facilities in local area, safety rating of area, problem rating of area; neighbourliness of area) (Model 5).

6 Health values score computed variable (Model 6).

7 Age (Model 7); sex (Model 8).

8 Socioeconomic status: variables measuring social class, personal total gross income, housing tenure, highest educational qualification) (Model 9).

These variables were either all statistically significant with bivariate analyses, or were considered as *a priori* hypotheses on the basis of the literature.

Table 3.1 presents the technical results of the final model, and these are summarized in Box 3.1. The table shows that the final model explained 25.9% (Adjusted R^2) of the variance in QoL ratings, and was highly significant ($p<0.001$; F statistic). The minus signs in the table indicate the direction of the question coding; all associations were in theoretically expected directions.

The nine models were each highly significant at $p<0.001$ (F values). The individual variables which retained significance in the final ninth model were social comparisons (Model 1), optimism-pessimism (in Model 2), health status and level of physical functioning (in Model 3), number of social activities, frequency of social contacts score, help and social support score, and the two items reflecting loneliness (in Model 4), ratings of the quality of the area (facilities) and safety ratings of the area (in Model 5), value for health (Model 6) and respondents' gender (Model 8). Neither the socioeconomic indicators (Model 9) nor the age of respondent (Model 7) were significant. The R^2 values for each of the nine models showed the amount of variance in QoL ratings explained by the variables. These are summarized in Box 3.1.

The total amount of explained variance, while only just over a quarter, is sizeable given the amorphous and subjective nature of the concept QoL. In sum, this suggests that the main independent predictors of self-rated global QoL, which explained over a quarter of the variance in QoL ratings (26.70%), were:

◆ *Social comparisons and expectations:* people's standards of social comparison and expectations in life (making downward comparisons of themselves with others less well off led people to rate their own QoL as better).

Table 3.1 Multiple regression of QoL rating

	Model 9 b
1 Social comparisons and expectations	
gap score[1]	−0.176
	−0.245 − −0.106
	(−4.97)***
2 Personality and psychology	
self-efficacy[2]	3.002E02
	−0.030 − 0.090
	(0.97)
Optimism-pessimism bias[2]	0.121
	0.030 − 0.212
	(2.61)**
Depression/anxiety (GHQ)[2]	1.060E02
	−0.016 − 0.037
	(0.79)
Self-assessed risks of negative life events[++1]	−4.649E03
	−0.067 − 0.058
	(−0.15)
3 Health	
Physical functioning (ADL score)[2]	6.709E02
	0.008 − 0.126
	(2.24)*
Health status[2]	0.209
	0.141 − 0.278
	(5.99)***
Long-standing illness[1]	3.699E02
	−0.090 − 0.164
	(0.57)
4 Social capital (personal)	
Social activities[1]	−0.118
	−0.191 − −0.045
	(−3.18)**
	(Continued)

Table 3.1 Continued

	Model 9 b
Social contacts[2]	−7.854E02
	−0.156−−0.001
	(−2.00)*
Social support[1]	−0.102
	−0.172−−0.032
	(−2.85)**
Pets[2]	−5.068E02
	−0.175−0.074
	(−0.80)
Frequency of loneliness[1]	−0.112
	−0.212−−0.013
	(−2.22)*
Increase in loneliness[1]	−0.152
	−0.263−−0.042
	(−2.72)**
5 Social capital	
Quality of area[2]	9.408E02
	0.029−0.159
	(2.85)**
Safety of area[2, +++]	0.101
	0.023−0.179
	(2.53)*
Problems of area[1]	3.787E02
	−0.025−0.101
	(1.18)
Neighbourliness of area[1]	5.653E02
	−0.057−0.170
	(0.97)
6 Health values	
Health value score[2]	−7.713E02
	−0.150−−0.004
	(−2.07)*

7 Age^2	3.014E03
	−0.007−−0.013
	(0.57)
8 Sex^1	−0.145
	−0.271−−0.018
	(−2.25)*
9 *Socioeconomic background*	
Social class^2	−3.432E02
	−0.082−0.014
	(−1.40)
Total income before tax^1	−8.911E03
	−0.020−0.002
	(−1.59)
Housing tenure^2	−2.895E02
	−0.093−0.035
	(−0.88)
Highest level of educational qualification^2	−2.174E02
	−0.051−0.007
	(−1.47)
Constant	3.739
R^2	0.290
Adjusted R^2	0.267
F statistic	12.78***
Change in adjusted R^2	0.010

Source: Bowling *et al.* (2002a)

The final (ninth) model shows that the percentage of total variation in QoL rating between groups which was explained by the model was 26.7 (Adjusted R^2)

No. of complete cases entered = 810

Variables within each model were entered in blocks

Multi-colinearity: all variables entered achieved correlations of less than 0.40

* $p<0.05$, ** $p<0.01$, *** $p<0.001$

Note: unstandardized coefficients and 95% confidence intervals displayed (2-tailed t values in parenthesis)

E-n = multiply by 10-n

1 Higher scores are better (female for RESPSEX)

2 Higher scores are worse (older for 'AGEGROUP' and no pets)

++ Excludes heart disease, cancer, housebound, memory loss, nursing home care

+++ Excludes 'never goes out' (63 people)

Box 3.1 Amount of explained variance in regression model of self-rated QoL

- Model 1 (social comparisons and expectations) explained 6.4% (Adjusted R^2) of the variance in QoL ratings.
- Adding in personality and psychological variables (Model 2) increased the amount of explained variation to 14.6%; these variables explained the most of the variance in QoL ratings (increasing the change in the adjusted R^2 by 8.2%).
- Adding health and functional status (Model 3) explained 20% of the variance (increasing the change in the adjusted R^2 by 5.4%).
- Adding personal social capital (social networks, support, activities) in Model 4 explained 23.1% of the variance (increasing the change in the adjusted R^2 by 3.1%).
- Adding external social capital (neighbourhood) (Model 5) explained 25.2% (increasing the change in the adjusted R^2 by 2.1%).
- Adding health values (Model 6) explained little at −25.5%. Adding age (Model 7) contributed nothing to the model (25.4%), and adding sex (Model 8) to the model, while it retained significance, explained little more (25.7%).
- Adding the socioeconomic indicators (Model 9) explained slightly more, 26.7%, of the variance in QoL ratings, but all lost significance.

- *Personality and psychological characteristics (optimism-pessimism):* a sense of optimism and belief that 'all will be well in the end' rather than a tendency to think the worst (or glass 'half full' rather than 'half empty' perspective on life).

- *Having good health and functional status.*

- *Personal social capital or resources:* engaging in a large number of social activities, having a higher level of social contacts, feeling helped and supported, low levels of loneliness.

- *External (neighbourhood) social capital:* living in a neighbourhood with perceived good quality community facilities and services, including transport, feeling safe in one's neighbourhood.

Self-efficacy did not retain significance in the final model. The effect of self-efficacy on QoL may have been mediating with functional status which did retain significance. These variables were consistent with the themes which emerged from the semi-structured and unstructured approaches (see next section), although income and self-efficacy did not retain statistical significance in the models, but need to be incorporated in a concept of QoL as they were included in the lay models.

Lay models of QoL

Research questions addressed in this survey were: how do older people perceive and prioritize their QoL? At the beginning of the interview respondents were asked open-ended questions about what were the good things that gave their lives quality, what were the bad things that took quality away, and how could QoL be improved?

Things that gave life quality

Analysis of respondents' views about what gave their lives quality revealed several key building blocks for a good QoL. In order of the frequency with which they were mentioned, these were: good social relationships (mentioned by 81%); having social roles and activities (60%); doing activities enjoyed alone (48%); having health (44%); psychological well-being (38%); living in a good home and neighbourhood (37%); adequacy of financial circumstances (33%); having independence and control over life (27%); society/politics (1%); other things (e.g. religion, having a good Christmas) were mentioned by 8%. These are shown in Table 3.2. Each of these main themes was also categorized by detailed sub-themes, which provided insight on how the theme mentioned affected people's quality of life (see Annex I for examples of these by theme).

It should be noted that, although religion was mentioned by just a few people in this study in terms of giving their life quality, this does not mean that it was not of relative importance to some people in other contexts. It is shown in Chapter 4 that 29% of all respondents had attended a place of worship in the past month. Religion has been reported to be salient to a number of older people in other studies (Browne *et al.* 1994; Koenig 1995). Those with belief have reported it to be important to their well-being in later life, especially when bereaved (Coleman *et al.* 2002), although larger population studies of widowed older people have found no associations between religious beliefs or philosophies and adjustment to widow(er)hood or loneliness (Bowling and Cartwright 1982).

Table 3.2 displays the main themes which were mentioned by survey respondents as giving quality to life, taking quality away from life, or either. There were differences in the QoL themes mentioned by age and sex of respondents. For

Table 3.2 Older people's definitions of the constituents of QoL (% survey respondents)+

Theme	Good things that give life quality++ % respondents	Bad things that take quality away from life++ % respondents	Mentioned theme as good or bad+++ % respondents
Social relationships	81	12	83
Social roles and activities	60	1	62
Other activities done alone	48	2	49
Health	44	50	76
Psychological factors	38	17	49
Home and neighbourhood	37	30	54
Financial circumstances	33	23	50
Independence	27	4	30
Other/miscellaneous	8	29	35
Society/politics	1	16	16
Number of respondents	**988**	**978**	**975**

Source: from a fuller table in Bowling et al. (2003). Reproduced with permission from Baywood Publishing Company Inc.
+ Open coding of survey responses.
++ Percentages total more than 100% as more than one theme could be mentioned (single, not multiple, responses per person within each theme only counted, and presented here).
+++ Base includes only people who mentioned both good and bad themes in order to give a common base number here.

example, reflecting traditional gender role divisions, women were more likely than men to mention home and neighbourhood, social relationships and social activities as giving their life quality, whereas men were more likely to mention finances and independence. And people aged 75+ were more likely than younger respondents to mention health, home and neighbourhood as giving life quality (for figures, and other associations, see later chapters on each theme).

It is important not to view these themes in isolation from each other. Respondents often commented on the subjectivity and multi-faceted nature of QoL, as well as the interdependent nature of its component parts. For example, having independence and social activities are often dependent on

Table 3.3 Older people's definitions of the constituents of QoL (in-depth interviews)+

Theme	Good things that give life quality % respondents	Bad things that take quality away from life % respondents	Mentioned theme as good or bad % respondents
Social relationships	96	80	99
Home and neighbourhood	96	84	100
Psychological factors	96	63	99
Other activities done alone	93	–	93
Health	85	83	99
Social roles and activities	80	1	80
Financial circumstances	73	53	91
Independence	69	46	84
Other/miscellaneous	18	19	31
Society/politics	1	43	43
Number of respondents	**80**	**80**	**80**

Source: from a fuller table in Bowling and Gabriel (2004). Reproduced with kind permission of Springer Science and Business Media.
+ As with Table 3.2, this table includes heterogeneous sub-groups: good only, bad only, good or bad themes mentioned (single counting only); and percentages total more than 100% as more than one theme could be mentioned (single responses within each theme presented here).

retaining good health and an adequate financial situation, as well as access to transport.

Table 3.3 shows that the same main themes were identified at the in-depth interviews with 80 of these survey respondents. The validity of the survey results in supported by comparable themes being identified. The difference is in the magnitude with which most of them were raised in the in-depth interviews; the larger proportions reflect the longer time respondents had to think and talk about the topic.

Things that took quality away from life

Survey respondents were asked what were the things that took quality away from their lives. Most, although not all, 'bad' quality of life areas which were mentioned were reversals of the 'good' themes (see Table 3.2). Poor health and functioning was most often mentioned (by 50%), followed by living in a bad home or neighbourhood (30%), inadequate finances (23%), poor psychological outlook (17%) and bad or inadequate social relationships (12%), loss of independence (4%), loss of social roles and activities (e.g. due to poor health), including those done alone such as reading (3%). Issues relating to wider society and politics were mentioned as bad areas of QoL (by 16%), rather than as good areas (1%). Particular reference was made here to government policies which were perceived to affect older people negatively (e.g. inadequate levels of state-funded pensions, inadequate policies to combat crime, immigration policies), as well as to negative world news which respondents said affected their mood adversely, pollution and environmental problems and policies, traffic and car-parking issues, local library closures, general concern about poor standards of behaviour in society, disrespectful or ageist attitudes and social values. Other 'bad' areas of QoL (mentioned by 29%) included reference to the poor British weather (cold, rain), and pressure to buy things by cold-callers (e.g. door-to-door salesmen) who were felt to target older people. Having a poor home and living in a bad neighbourhood, poor health and poor social relationships were most often mentioned by in-depth sample members as the things that took quality away from their lives (see Table 3.3).

Single most important aspect of QoL

Respondents were asked which of the areas of QoL they had mentioned was the *single* most important to them. The two most frequently mentioned important areas were having good social relationships (e.g. having a good family/marriage/friends and neighbours, and pets) (mentioned by 37%) and having good health (37%). People who were widowed or divorced/separated were the groups most likely to say social relationships were the most important, again suggesting that people valued what they had lost (45% and 42% respectively), in comparison with those who were married (35%), cohabiting (30%) or single (13%). Some people included their pets here, regarding them as part of their families, for example, one woman who derived a great deal of comfort and companionship from her pet dog, said: 'The most important to me are my family and my dog – I don't know which one I would put first, as the dog is family.'

Health was frequently said to be essential for the other aspects of life, as these two people said: 'Good health is needed to be able to carry on with the other activities I do.' 'You can't buy health, health must be the main source of satisfaction and happiness.' There were no significant associations with health and physical functioning and the people who mentioned, or did not mention, this theme.

Other areas prioritized, but by far fewer people (2–6% in each category) included maintaining independence (being able to do things for themselves and continue with their social activities), having a good home and living in a good neighbourhood, having a positive outlook (psychological well-being), having enough money, having social roles and activities, including solitary activities (e.g. knitting, reading), society/politics (e.g. government policy on pensions or other areas which affected people's well-being).

Improving QoL for themselves

Following their self-ratings of QoL, respondents were then asked what single thing would improve the quality of their lives. The most common responses were having better health and physical mobility (some also mentioned the need for better health care) (34%), having more money/a bigger pension (30%), followed by having better social relationships with family members or friends/neighbours (although this was by fewer, 9%).

Respondents who reported having a long-standing illness were more likely than those who did not report this to mention having good health as the single area which would most improve their quality of life: 44% and 17% respectively. Again, those with severe, or great, difficulties with activities of daily living were more likely to mention having their health as the single area that would give quality to their lives: 59% and 54% respectively, compared with 39% with moderate, 32% with slight and 21% of those with no difficulties.

There was a significant association between reported loneliness and mentioning better social relationships as the single thing that would improve their quality of life: 37% of those who said they 'always' felt lonely, and 27% of those who said they 'often' felt lonely mentioned social relationships in this context, in comparison with fewer of those who said they 'sometimes' felt lonely (11%) and those who said they 'never' felt lonely (5%). Some respondents suggested how they might be helped: 'I'd like a friend, someone I could trust.' 'Living with someone to avoid loneliness.' 'My family living closer.'

Respondents on the lowest incomes were the most likely to say that more money would improve their own quality of life: 35% of those receiving less than £4160 said this, as did 32% receiving £4160<£9360, compared with fewer, 23%, of those with £9360<£17,680 and 23% of those with £17,680+. As one man said: 'If people could have about £100 per week on top of bills – sometimes there is something I would like, such as a regular holiday, or trips – more money to go out for the day and perhaps buy lunch out . . . I get just over £101 per week, but when you take the rent and council tax off I end up with about £50 for everything.'

Other areas were mentioned by less than 7%: living in a better home or area, having their independence (e.g. being able to drive again, to be able to get out and about), more social roles and activities (including solo activities), having a more positive disposition and society/politics (e.g. government policies on pensions, crime). Some people mentioned practical things: 'To have no stairs.' 'A wee bit more money to build a downstairs toilet.' 'Transport – accessible to people with disabilities, level access at each stop.' 'Knowing that it is safe to go out and about.' 'To get involved in something, to be part of something.'

The most commonly mentioned things that in-depth interview respondents said would improve the quality of their lives were having a better home and neighbourhood (mentioned by 33%), having enough money (30%) and better health (25%).

Improving QoL for older people in general

Finally, respondents were then asked what *single* thing would improve the overall quality of life for *people of their age*. The two most common responses again were to have enough money, better financial circumstances or higher pensions (44%), followed by better health (some of these also said better health care) (27%). A few mentioned home and neighbourhood, social relationships, roles and activities, psychological well-being, independence and society/politics (<10% in each case).

There were no significant associations with sociodemographic, social or psychological characteristics or circumstances and those who mentioned, or did not mention, these themes, except with reported loneliness and mentioning social relationships as the most important thing that would improve other people's quality of life: 25% of those who said they 'always' felt lonely mentioned this, in comparison with 8–9% respectively of those who said they 'often' or 'sometimes' felt lonely, and 5% of those who said they never felt lonely. A poignant comment was made by one respondent in relation to the distance between many families: 'If we could be friends with our own families and keep in touch.'

However, a few said that social inclusion was an issue for wider society: 'Greater inclusion of the elderly in society if they wanted.' 'Greater tolerance of the aged by the younger generation.' Some people also said there was still a need for cheaper public transport and more security (personal safety) to enable people to feel confident going out, especially at night, which also has implications for maintaining social activities and contacts.

In sum, the analysis of the open-ended survey responses and the responses to the in-depth interviews illustrated that people's definitions generally corresponded with the theoretical definitions and models presented earlier, although in far greater detail. But the model of QoL stemming from this research needs supplementing with the two additional areas emphasized by older people themselves: the importance of the perception of having an adequate income, and of retaining independence and control over one's life.

Moreover, some of the more detailed sub-themes identified by respondents in both the open-ended survey questions and in-depth interviews have received little emphasis in the theoretical or practical literature (e.g. the benefits of lack of time constraints in retirement, enjoyment of one's home, the importance of the wider community and social capital, the necessity of being able to drive, and to afford to maintain, and run, a car for maintenance of independence and enjoyment of life in older age – see later chapters).

Conclusion

Most people rated their QoL at the good end of the scale, although there was a trend with age with almost three-quarters of the group aged 65–69 rating their lives overall as 'So good it could not be better' or 'Very good' in comparison with about half to a third of those in older age groups. However, age did not retain significance in the regression model as an independent predictor of ratings of life quality. Sex emerged as significant in the model, but explained very little of the variation in QoL ratings.

A lay model of QoL emerged from respondents' descriptions of the quality of their lives. The main themes which emerged from both the open-ended survey responses and the in-depth, follow-up interviews overlapped considerably: social relationships, social roles and activities, other activities enjoyed alone, health, home and neighbourhood, psychological well-being, financial circumstances, independence. Society/political issues were mentioned more in relation to factors which took quality away from their lives (e.g. government policies). The difference was simply in the magnitude with which these themes were mentioned between these analyses (i.e. most in-depth interviewees mentioned each theme, reflecting the greater length of time given to exploring topics, whilst there was more variation among the survey respondents). There were differences by age and sex of respondent and the type of themes mentioned, with the associations by sex partly reflecting traditional gender role divisions in society.

The quantitative regression model overlapped considerably with the lay models, except that self-efficacy (a measure of self-mastery and control over the important things in life) and socioeconomic factors, including finances, did not retain their earlier significance in the model. But respondents to the open-ended survey questions and to the in-depth interviews emphasized the importance of retaining their independence and control over life in older age, as well as having enough money.

It is possible that the measure of self-efficacy was either mediating between variables or it was insensitive to issues of independence and control over life in older age, with the implication that, as people themselves say that this area is important for QoL, improved measures are needed. One indicator which enables independence and control over life, apart from self-efficacy, is functional ability. Health and functioning were indeed significant, independent predictors of perceived QoL. However, having enough money is also an enabling factor. In relation to the results on finances, it is possible that, in older age when incomes are more levelled due to people's reliance mainly on pensions (although a wide range of annual income still exists), objective indicators of financial status are less sensitive than perceived financial circumstances. This finding also has implications for the design of measurement instruments (i.e. perceptions are important to tap).

Using this multi-method approach, the main themes which emerged as the drivers of QoL, thus forming its foundations, are summarized below:

- good social relationships with family, friends and neighbours;
- good home and neighbourhood (safe, good facilities including transport);
- positive outlook and psychological well-being;
- activities/hobbies (enjoyed alone);
- good health and functional ability;
- social roles and engaging in social and voluntary activities (with others);
- adequate income;
- independence and control over one's life.

These data are supported by wider European surveys about the main concerns of older people, in which health, independence, relationships, loneliness, money and neighbourhood safety feature prominently (Pfizer 2002). In particular, the psychological characteristics of optimism-pessimism explained the greatest amount of the variance in the quantitative regression model, and psychological outlook and well-being were also among the most frequently mentioned areas of QoL in the in-depth interviews. It was the sixth most frequently mentioned theme in the open-ended survey responses. This suggests that QoL is strongly influenced by psychological outlook, in support of the increasingly popular psychological theories of well-being and life quality (see Chapter 1).

In conclusion, the respondents to the QoL survey reported here emphasized the importance of having good social relationships and contacts, retaining their social roles and activities (including those hobbies and leisure activities enjoyed alone), having their health and physical ability, living in a good home and neighbourhood, adopting a positive psychological outlook and good psychological well-being, having enough money, and remaining independence as giving life quality ('good' areas). Most respondents mentioned several areas of life as making up the QoL, and commented on the subjectivity and multi-faceted nature of QoL, as well as the interdependent nature of its component parts. For example, having good health and physical functioning is necessary for maintaining social roles and activities. The following chapters in this book expand on the main themes mentioned, and which contributed most to perceived QoL.

Annex I: Summary of sub-themes: older people's models of good and bad quality of life

Social relationships (good)
◆ has partner;
◆ has good relationships (close/loving/caring/supportive/someone to love);
◆ has family to do things with;
◆ sees family;
◆ has contact with (great) grandchildren;
◆ enjoys sharing other people's children;
◆ enjoys seeing family happy/achieve/progress;
◆ has contact with family by phone/post;
◆ has practical help/regular help from family (e.g. with shopping, housework, bathing, gardening);
◆ feels secure knowing family would help if needed;
◆ gives practical help/support to friends/neighbours/family members;
◆ has good, reciprocal relationship with family/friends/neighbours;

- sees friends;
- has good/close friends;
- has friends to do things with;
- has practical help from friends;
- has telephone contact with friends;
- has company (for mixing, conversation/to be nice to one);
- has pet for company/to love/to depend on them.

Social relationships (bad)

- misses spouse who died (for compatibility/love/familiarity/help with practical tasks/shared decision-making/responsibility);
- misses friends/family members (not spouse) who have died;
- poor relationships (e.g. fallen out with others/unhappy family/quarrels between other family members);
- has no family to do things with/go out with/go on holiday with;
- does not see family enough;
- family too busy to visit/spend time with one;
- lack of satisfactory contact with family by phone/post;
- lack of contact with (great) grandchildren;
- family would/could not help if needed;
- has no friends to do things with;
- has no good/close friends;
- does not see friends;
- has no practical help from friends;
- lack of satisfactory contact with friends by phone;
- friends too busy to help/spend time with one;
- has no company (e.g. for mixing/conversation/to be nice to one).

Social roles and social activities (good only)

- helps friends, family, neighbours (e.g. child care, collecting things from shops);
- does voluntary work;
- committee member of local group;
- performs in arts, drama, music group/choir;
- attends local events/meetings/education classes;
- attends age-related clubs;
- has holidays/weekends away;
- goes on outings/day trips/shopping with someone else;
- has meals/drinks out;
- gambles (e.g. horses, bingo);
- goes to cultural events (e.g. theatre/concerts/cinema);
- attends place of worship;
- mental pursuits to keep mind alert (evening classes, quizzes, bridge);

- does sports/exercises/dancing activities;
- walking dog – helps to meet others/caring for pet.

Solo activities (alone) – mostly good

- crafts including woodwork, embroidery, restoring antiques, sewing, knitting, crochet, painting, flower arranging;
- hobbies including stamp, coin, book or other types of collecting;
- maintaining cultural interest in art/theatre/architecture;
- technical hobbies including photography, videoing;
- home improvement activities (DIY);
- cooking/eating new foods/new diet;
- having a drink at home;
- watching sport on TV;
- listening to music on audio-cassettes/radio/watching TV/videos;
- playing an instrument alone (e.g. piano, organ);
- reading books, poetry;
- reading newspapers/keeping up to date with current affairs;
- mental pursuits including doing crosswords, jigsaws, competitions, writing;
- gardening or tending allotment, caring for indoor plants;
- watching wildlife (e.g. feeding and watching birds, badgers, squirrels, foxes, butterflies);
- doing (solitary) physical activities, exercise, keeping fit, walking, jogging, walking the dog for exercise.

Health (good)

- good health relative to others/self in past (i.e. downward health comparison with those who are worse off, or oneself in the past when worse off (i.e. 'before medical/surgical intervention'));
- having health;
- access to good health care;
- coping with health condition: makes the best of things; able to do things despite health problem;
- fit enough to do what one wants/general activities/social activities/go out as much as wants/do hobbies/play with grandchildren;
- still able to drive due to having health.

Health (poor)

- poor health relative to others/self in past (i.e. upwards health comparison with those who are better off healthwise, or self in the past when better off healthwise);
- losing health;
- access to poor health care;
- discomfort due to restricted functioning (e.g. when stretching, bending, using stairs, sitting, standing, kneeling, balancing);

- not fit enough to do what one wants/general activities/social activities/go out as much as wants/do hobbies/play with grandchildren;
- unable to drive due to poor health;
- difficulties looking after self and home (e.g. bathing, housework, shopping, gardening);
- difficulties communicating (e.g. poor hearing on telephone);
- pain/aches/other symptoms;
- tiredness/lack of energy;
- restrictions on diet;
- close other's poor health.

Psychological outlook and well-being (good)
- enjoys life;
- enjoys having social role;
- enjoys being busy;
- mentally alert;
- derives psychological strength to face future from spiritual/religious beliefs;
- positive disposition (happy, content, outlook 'make own quality of life');
- positive memories of past (work, achievements, family);
- self-confident;
- enthusiasm for future, looks forward to things;
- stress-free;
- not lonely;
- feels lucky;
- feels good about having healthy lifestyle;
- ability to cope with bad things;
- feels good – achieving goals, able to do what wants to.

Psychological outlook and well-being (bad)
- does not enjoy life;
- unhappy due to lack of social role;
- unhappy as not busy/occupied;
- unhappy/depressed as not come to terms with spouse's death;
- unhappy – no emotional support;
- memory deteriorating;
- no psychological strength from religious beliefs;
- negative disposition (depressed, unhappy, discontent);
- negative memories of past (work, achievements, family);
- loss of confidence due to poor health, poor family relationships, poor neighbourhood;
- lack of enthusiasm for future, does not look forward to things;
- stressed;
- lonely;
- feels unlucky;

- unable to cope with bad things;
- feels bad – not achieving goals, not able to do what wants to;
- feels bad about unhealthy lifestyle.

Home and neighbourhood (good)

- likes living alone;
- pleasant landscape/surroundings;
- friendly area/community feel;
- feels safe/secure;
- good public transport;
- good local services (e.g. council, police, repairs, street lights, refuse);
- good library/mobile library service;
- good local facilities (e.g. shops/post-office/market);
- lives near family;
- good relationships with neighbours;
- enjoys/derives pleasure from home (e.g. comfortable/spacious/nice).

Home and neighbourhood (bad)

- dislikes living alone;
- unpleasant surroundings;
- unfriendly area/no community feel;
- feels unsafe (e.g. fear of crime, being attacked/going out at night/damage to property/ burglaries);
- poor public transport;
- poor local services (e.g. council, police, repairs, street lights, refuse);
- poor library/mobile library service;
- poor local facilities (e.g. shops/post-office/market);
- lives far away from family;
- poor relationship with neighbours;
- stressed by home (e.g. repairs needed/stairs/household chores difficult).

Financial circumstances (good)

- adequate income/pension;
- adequate income/pension/standard of living due to low financial expectations – perceived to be adequate relative to others/parent/self in past/in comparison with what expected (e.g. downward wealth comparison with those who are worse off in some way, or oneself in the past when worse off);
- solvent, able to pay for basics, to afford essentials and pay basic bills (e.g. heating, balanced diet, clothes, telephone);
- able to afford to run/maintain car/petrol;
- able to afford to pay for help with everyday tasks in the home/upkeep or repairs to house;

- able to afford to pursue luxuries including hobbies, pastimes, pets, travel, have holidays;
- Home ownership.

Financial circumstances (bad)
- inadequate income/pension;
- not solvent, unable to pay bills, has debts;
- no longer able to afford to run/maintain car/petrol;
- not able to afford to pay for help with everyday tasks in the home/upkeep or repairs to house;
- not able to afford luxuries or to pursue hobbies/pastimes/pets, travel, have holidays.

Independence (has)
- able to do things for self (e.g. looking after home, garden) makes one happy, good mood;
- fit enough to retain independence;
- can please self, no one else to consider (e.g. widowed);
- independent due to lack of restrictions on time/flexibility of time when retired (e.g. to do things one wants/take holidays/hobbies/shopping/time get up);
- independent due to having health – going out/away;
- independent due to being healthy enough to drive car;
- independent due to being able to afford to run car (maintenance, petrol).

Independence (lost)
- unable to do things for self – leads to depression/frustration;
- not fit enough to be independent (e.g. with looking after self/home);
- unable to drive car due to health limitations (coded here where led to loss of independence);
- unable to drive car as much as wants to cost of petrol/car maintenance (coded here where led to loss of independence);
- unable to please self/do what one wants (e.g. limitations other/(ill) spouse to consider).

Global society and politics (mostly bad)
- depressed by negative world news;
- concern about poor values/standards of behaviour in society in general/ageist attitudes;
- perception of high crime rates in society in general;
- disagreement with government policies – including pensions, Europe, immigration, ageist policies.

4

Social relationships and activities

The quality of my life now is my family – my children and grandchildren. My life surrounds them.

So, helping people does . . . help your own quality of life . . . it gives me such a lot of pleasure . . .

. . . Mine [QoL] is to get out and about . . . or see things that I would like to see or haven't seen.

Social relationships

It was pointed out in Chapter 1 that, despite inconsistencies, fairly strong evidence appears to exist between high levels of social support and reduction of mortality risk, improved mental and physical health status, physical performance and well-being (Berkman and Syme 1979; Blazer 1982; House et al. 1988; Olsen 1992; Bowling 1994; Seeman et al. 1996a, 1996b, 2001; Strawbridge et al. 1996; Bowling and Grundy 1998; Stansfeld 1999). There is evidence that this health benefit remains influential in very old age (Grundy et al. 1996). Marriage has also been positively linked to health, and divorce and widow(er)hood can have a negative impact on health and longevity, particularly for men (Bowling 1987, 1988; Bowling and Charlton 1987; Verbrugge 1989).

Much of this literature indicates that social relationships and activity *per se* appear to confer health benefits through psychosocial pathways. In support of this, there are long-established associations between social participation and/ or support and feelings of security, self-esteem and hence self-mastery, especially if relationships are reciprocal (Lawton 1980; Wentowski 1981; Wenger 1992). On the other hand, health status and functional ability have also been reported to contribute more to the life satisfaction of older people than social networks or support (Bowling and Browne 1991; Bowling et al. 1991). The research linking social support to life satisfaction and well-being in older age is not all consistent, probably reflecting the wide range of measures, of varying quality, employed. But an emphasis on social health is supported by research on the public's priorities in life, which has reported that social relationships and activities are among the most important areas of life nominated by the public, and a main area that gives quality to life (Bowling 1995a, 1995b; Farquhar 1995; Bowling and Windsor 2001; Bowling et al. 2003; see also Chapter 3). The importance of social networks lies in the extent to which they provide help and support. Social support involves emotional concern (feeling liked, loved, esteemed); instrumental aid (services); information (about environment); and appraisal (information for self-evaluation) (Cobb 1976; House 1981; Thoits 1982). Thus support exists only if it leads to certain beliefs in the recipient. The structural characteristics of the network influence the availability and perceived adequacy of help and support from network members (Mitchell 1969; Craven and Wellman 1974; Walker et al. 1997).

The percentage of older people who live alone is much higher in western developed nations than in eastern and southern developed and developing counties (Grundy and Bowling 1997). And while in pre-industrial Britain more older people lived with their children than today, this was mainly because elderly people were more likely to have an unmarried child living at home. The trend towards residential independence with older age since the last half of the twentieth century, with older people increasingly living alone or with their partners only, reflects not so much that families do not provide support for their older members, but that independence is a preferred norm. In the post-war years relationships with family certainly played a central theme in the lives of older people in Britain (Townsend 1957; Young and Wilmott 1957), although friendships may have increased in importance since, with the decline of the extended family. However, deteriorations in the social networks of older people are likely to have been exaggerated. National data for Britain indicates that the vast majority of older people have at least weekly contact with relatives and neighbours, although contact with friends was less frequent. And those in the manual social classes were more likely than those in the non-manual classes to have daily face-to-face contact with relatives, and to have relatives living nearby (Coulthard et al. 2001; Office for National Statistics 2004). The social networks of most older people still consist mainly of relatives, and these kin provide most of the instrumental help required, but having friends, and in particular a confidant, is important for the emotional well-being and self-esteem of older people (Blau 1973; Wenger 1984a; and see Bowling 1991, 1994; Bowling and Grundy 1998).

Social activity

On retirement from paid work, people are released from the structure and constraints that it placed on their lives. Leisure time is increased, and people can, in theory, spend their time as they wish. Participation in a wide range of social and community activities comprises an area where older people can make a significant contribution to their local community. Social activities can also provide older people with opportunities to maintain and expand a circle of friends and acquaintances, and acquire new partners after widow(er)hood. An ability to participate in leisure and social activities is likely to be important to QoL. Getting out and about, and maintaining social contact, is an important activity for all people, but can be particularly important for those older people who live more isolated lives. Rowe and Kahn (1998) argued that engagement with life, along with avoidance of disease and maintenance of physical and cognitive functioning is a critical component of successful ageing. Initially formulated as activity theory (see Chapter 1), this perspective proposes that greater social activity and participation compensates for the role loss which accompanies retirement and older age (Havighurst et al. 1968). Atchley (1989) later revised this theory, shifting the emphasis away from the volume of activities and stressed adjustment to ageing via the substitution and redistribution of activities. While criticized for failing to adequately consider the circumstances of very frail and ill people, this 'resilience', as a result of the ability to compensate for the erosion of skills to perform essential activities, was stressed by Baltes and Baltes (1990b) in their theories of ageing well. Of course, such components are interdependent – having good health and functioning enhances one's ability to maintain social activities (Rowe and Kahn 1998).

Engaging in leisure activities has been associated with positive outcome in later life in a number of studies, including associations with reduction in mortality risk (e.g. Kaplan et al. 1996; Glass et al. 1999), reduced risk of cognitive impairment (Fabrigoule et al. 1995; Wang et al. 2002), improved physical health (Menec and Chipperfield 1997) and older people's perceptions that their lives have improved (Silverstein and Parker 2002). Occupying several social roles, including membership of clubs and associations, has been positively associated with health and longevity (Berkman and Breslow 1983; House et al. 1988; Moen et al. 1989). Role accumulation, as a compensatory strategy, may be particularly important in later life when the chances of role loss increase. One strategy that some older people use when retired from paid work is engaging in voluntary work, and they have been reported to find this satisfying, as well as a source of new social contacts and friends (Boaz et al. 1999). A review of the literature by Boaz et al. on the attitudes of a wide sample of people aged 50 and over in the UK reported that overall respondents expressed a high degree of satisfaction with their social activities, and wanted to be socially active.

However, the ability to make full use of personal freedom in older age is partly dependent on financial status, health and physical mobility, place of residence and the social capital of the local area. Other limitations include family commitments, including the constraints associated with being a carer. More than one in five people aged 50 and over in England and Wales provide unpaid care for family members, friends or relatives. While the proportion declines with age, this still leaves 5% of people aged 85+ providing such care (Office for National Statistics 2004). Membership of informal organizations is also class-related. For example, analyses of the British Household Panel Survey for 1999 found that overall a majority of middle-class older men, but only a minority of working-class older men, were members of at least one informal organization (Davidson et al. 2002). Moreover, population data show that people aged 65 and over in the UK spend more time than those aged 50–64 in sedentary activities such as watching television, listening to the radio or to music, or reading, and also more time resting or 'doing nothing special', possibly due to barriers to more active pursuits, including poorer health and mobility, poor transport and lower income (Office for National Statistics 2004).

The survey

This section is divided into two parts. In the first, the results for social relationships are presented, followed by social activities in the second. The questions on social network and support included items from questionnaires developed for the British General Household Survey, some of which were also derived from Rand's Social Support Scale (Sherbourne and Stewart 1991; Coulthard et al. 2001; Walker et al. 2001). These were supplemented by questions on type of different social activities engaged in over the past month, and ratings of their importance to respondents.

Social relationships

As would be expected from national data, almost two-thirds of respondents were married or cohabiting and about a third of respondents lived alone (see

---

Box 4.1 Social network structures

- 86% said they had a son or daughter still alive.
- Of these, 62% said their children lived within five miles of them (including same household).
- 73% had live brothers and sisters. Of these, just 36% said their siblings lived within five miles.
- 59% of all respondents said they had a relative whom they felt 'close to' living near by.
- 74% said they had 'close friends' who lived near by.
- 7% said they had a pet (mainly a dog, cat or bird).

Chapter 2). The vast majority of respondents reported having their children or close friends living near to them, although this still left substantial minorities who did not. More people reported having 'close friends' than 'close relatives' living nearby (see Box 4.1).

Frequency of social contacts

While most respondents had at least weekly face-to-face and telephone contacts with friends and relatives, this again leaves a substantial minority – about four in ten people – who had a low frequency of social contacts, and who were at risk of isolation (see Box 4.2). Number of contacts was not associated with socioeconomic indicators.

Contact with relatives and friends by letter was infrequent, with 27% reporting sending or receiving such letters at least monthly, and for the remainder it was less often than this or not at all. Email was not used to substitute or supplement contacts – 90% did not use email for contact with relatives and friends.

Box 4.2 Social contacts

- 62% saw relatives face-to-face at least weekly.
- 81% had daily to more than weekly contact with relatives by phone.
- 72% saw friends face-to-face at least weekly.
- 64% had daily to more than weekly contact with friends by phone.
- 19% had a high frequency of social contact score (e.g. daily contacts with relatives and/or friends), 40% had a middle score and 41% had a low score.

Most respondents believed that they could command help and support when needed. They were asked whether they could turn to someone for practical help in a range of situations (needing a lift urgently, help needed when ill in bed, financial difficulties, everyday chores) and between 79% and 95% said they could (see Box 4.3). Relatives were the most commonly mentioned as the people they would call for help. It is well known from other research that families, particularly daughters, provide the most practical help for older people, often at the cost of considerable stress to themselves (see Bowling 1991, 1994 for review).

Almost everyone said they could call on someone for emotional support. Whether they actually would is unknown, but this figure appears high, especially when compared with the percentage who said they were lonely (see p. 98). This high estimation of help and support has been reported in similar studies of older people (Grundy and Bowling 1999). It is possible that some social desirability bias (the wish to present a positive image of oneself) operates with these questions.

While there were no differences with gender, there were some differences with age group, with older respondents being the most vulnerable. People aged 75+ were less likely than those aged <75 to say they had someone to provide help, possibly reflecting the greater number of bereavements of friends and relatives that are experienced with older age. For example, 95% of those aged <75 had someone they could ask for a lift, and 86% of those aged 75+ had someone. And both men and women aged 75+ were also significantly less likely than those aged <75 to say they had someone they could ask for financial help: 83% of those aged <75 and 73% of those 75+ said they had someone.

Similarly, while there were no differences with gender and *actual number* of practical areas of life one could ask for help with (help with a lift, help

---

Box 4.3 Help and support

Has someone to ask for help when:

- Need someone for comfort or support in a crisis (99%)
- Ill in bed and needed help (96%)
- Need a lift urgently (91%)
- Need help with everyday tasks (91%)
- In financial difficulties (79%)

---

when ill, help with finances and everyday tasks), both men and women aged 75+ were less likely than people aged <75 to have someone who could help in three or four (as opposed to one or two) of these four areas: 76% of those aged <75 and 63% of those aged 75+ could ask for help in all areas. As indicated above, some decline in help is perhaps inevitable, given that the illnesses and deaths of friends and relatives become more common with increasing age. But it is possible that personality is also an influencing factor here. It is reported in Chapter 6 that high self-efficacy appeared to be an enabling characteristic, and was associated with having more areas of life one could ask for help with. This supports psychological theories of QoL (see Chapter 1).

Help can also be reciprocal, and older people can be providers of help and support, as well as receiving it. US approaches to exchange theory postulate that successful relationships depend on each participant trying to get what they need by exchanging valued resources with others having resources to deploy (Blau 1964). Older people are disadvantaged in this model, as they are often regarded as having few resources to exchange. However, modifications of exchange theory postulate that, by participating in relationships based on mutual loyalty and sharing, older, as well as younger, people can make contributions to, and derive benefits from, interactions with people and the wider social system. For example, as is shown in the section on social activities, just under a fifth, 17%, of respondents said that, in the past month, they had looked after someone who is ill or frail, and about a quarter, 24%, had baby-sat or child-minded. Data from the USA also shows that even among people aged 75+ with functional limitations, most report that they give as much support to their families as they receive (Antonucci and Jackson 1989).

Aloneness and loneliness

About six in ten of the respondents (59%) lived with their spouses or partner only, and three in ten lived alone, reflecting national statistics (Walker *et al.* 2001). Of the remainder, four people lived with their spouse plus a son or daughter and three lived with a son or daughter only. A sizeable minority of people also said they spent a great deal of time alone (see over leaf). Time spent alone is not, in itself, an index of social isolation, especially when many people live alone, but it can be a marker for vulnerability when people also feel lonely. A third of elderly people were relatively solitary, and over a third were lonely:

- 35% said they were 'Often' or 'Always' alone, the remainder said 'Seldom' or 'Never';

- 34% said they spent more, rather than less or the same, amount of time alone than ten years ago;

- 7% said they 'Always' or 'Often' felt lonely; 32% were 'Sometimes' lonely, the remainder said they were 'Never' lonely.

While the percentage who said they felt lonely 'Sometimes' (32%) was higher than figures from early, classic studies conducted between 1948 and 1968 (13–25%), the percentages who reported that they were 'Always' lonely were very similar across these studies (Victor *et al.* 2004), indicating little substantial change. The amount of time spent alone was associated with loneliness. Three-quarters of those who said they were 'Seldom' or 'Never' alone also said they 'Never' felt lonely. In comparison, a little over a third (37%) of those who said they were 'Always' or 'Often' alone said they 'Never' felt lonely. Having a pet made no difference to reporting loneliness. And while living alone should not necessarily be equated with social isolation, given that social network members can live in proximity, people who lived with others were far more likely to say they 'Never' felt lonely – 85% in comparison with 32% of those who lived alone who said this. Men were more likely than women, especially older women (aged 75+), to report that they were 'Never' lonely: 71% of males and 51% of females said this. It is unknown whether this partly reflects gender differences in willingness to admit to, and report, feelings.

And while people can, of course, be lonely within married relationships, married people were less likely to report loneliness. Respondents who were married or cohabiting were the most likely to report that they were 'Never lonely' – 78% said this, in comparison with 49% of those who were single, 49% of those who were divorced or separated and 29% of those who were widowed. The literature has long indicated that loneliness is a particular problem for widowed people, especially as they are no longer the object of a spouse's love and attention, and not just because of their loss of activities engaged in as a couple (Townsend 1957; Tunstall 1966; Bowling and Cartwright 1982).

Victor *et al.* (2004) reported in more detail on the main risk factors for loneliness among sample members, which included being unmarried, as well as being in poor physical and mental health. These associations with health were consistent with earlier research by Bowling *et al.* (1989). While older age appeared to protect against loneliness, they identified six major factors, independent of each other, which increased older people's vulnerability to the risk of loneliness: being unmarried, amount of time spent alone, reported increases in loneliness, psychological morbidity and poor psychological and physical health.

Associations with QoL

Associations with QoL ratings   Table 4.1 displays dichotomized QoL ratings for simplicity of presentation. These show that respondents who could ask for practical help with the most things (apart from an inconsistency at the lower end of the scale), who had someone they could turn to for comfort (most people reported having someone, reducing the sensitivity of this variable), and who reported the most social activities (and see p. 108), were more likely than other respondents to rate the quality of their lives as good. There were no associations with frequency of social contacts (relatives and friends combined). More detailed breakdowns have been reported elsewhere (see Bowling *et al.* 2002a).

In addition (not shown in the table), people who were married or cohabiting rated their QoL as highest: 55% of those who were married or cohabiting said their QoL was 'So good it could not be better' or 'Very good', in comparison with 45% of those who were widowed, 44% of those who were divorced or separated and 33% of those who were single. And feeling isolated (being 'Always' or 'Often' alone), lonely and feeling more lonely than ten years ago were also all associated with worse QoL self-ratings. For example, 42% of those who 'Always', 'Often' or 'Sometimes' felt lonely, rated their QoL as 'So good could not be better' to 'Very good', in comparison with 55% who 'Never' felt lonely.

Finally, social network and support factors were significant independent predictors of self-rated overall QoL. It was shown in Chapter 3 that adding personal social capital (social contacts, support, loneliness, social activities) into the regression model of independent predictors of self-rated QoL increased the change in the adjusted R^2 by a small but significant amount – 3.1%.

Lay models

Things that gave life quality

Social relationships was the most common thing that respondents mentioned gave their lives quality (81%) ('good' QoL). It was also mentioned by almost all (96%) of the in-depth interview respondents as giving life quality (see Annex I for a summary of the sub-themes).

As was expected from earlier research by the author (Bowling 1995a, 1995b; Bowling and Windsor 2001; Bowling *et al.* 2003), women were more likely than

Table 4.1 Respondents' social network, support and activity characteristics by QoL rating (row %)

Social network, support and activity characteristics	QoL rating (row %)	
	So good it could not be better/very good/good	Alright/bad/very bad/so bad it could not be worse
Practical support score (no. of areas can ask for practical help with) ('PRACHELP') (n = 992)		
0	61	39***
1	45	55
2	69	31
3	77	23
4	86	14
Has someone to turn to for comfort/ support in personal crisis ('COMFORT') (n = 987)		
1+ people	82	18***
No one	58	42
Frequency of contact with relatives and friends score ('SOCTOT') (n = 992)		
< 26 (high)	76	24 ±
26–30	85	15
31–51 (low)	82	18
Number of different social activities score ('ACTIVTOT') (n = 993):		
0	53	46***
1–2	74	26
3–4	85	15
5+	91	9

*** p<0.001, ± not statistically significant (chi-square test)

men to say that relationships gave their life quality: 89% compared with 72% of men. There were no associations with age or social class. But people who had experienced a married relationship were also more likely to mention social relationships as making up a good QoL: that is, 89% of those who were widowed, 78% of those who were married or cohabiting and 73% of those who were divorced/separated mentioned social relationships, in comparison with fewer single people and people who were cohabiting (66% and 67% respectively, mentioned this theme). This suggests that people valued the intimate relationships that they had, and those which they had lost through being widowed, divorced or separated. Reported loneliness did not show any consistent pattern with mentioning social relationships as making up a good QoL.

Consistent with the literature on social support and well-being (see Chapter 1), social relationships with family, friends and neighbours were important to people for companionship, people to do things with (going out, going on holidays), to help practically, to feel cared for, to prevent loneliness and to promote psychological well-being. Respondents referred to the importance of having a good, close, supportive, loving relationship with their family; and those who were married mentioned the importance of having a good, compatible, loving and familiar relationship with their partner. Respondents emphasized the importance of having someone for 'companionship', to 'take me out', 'to be nice to me', 'to make life bearable', to 'know there is someone there willing to help me' or 'look after me'.

Meaningful contact, face to face or by telephone, with sons and daughters was important to most respondents for enjoyment, help and security. Some respondents commented that having someone nearby, to call on for help, also gave them confidence. Relatives were seen as more likely than friends to provide this support. Friendships are voluntary relationships, in contrast to the traditional role obligations involved in familial relationships; they are based on emotional domains, and may have difficulty withstanding the demands of long-term care provision (Johnson 1983). One woman distinguished clearly between the types of people one could call on for help:

R: I have a daughter who lives about 10 minutes away . . . so I see her frequently. So I have her to hand, as it were, absolutely.
I: OK. And do you think that affects the quality of life?
R: Oh yes, definitely. Definitely, yes. It's um [*short pause*] you know, always somebody I can call on in, if there's a necessity so to do . . . I can call upon my daughter . . . Um, which I am sure enhances my quality of life, because I think . . . friends are very good friends, but you can't call upon people unless you know them terribly

well, to take you to the [hospital] for a test. You know, those sorts of things, you really need family for that.

(Mrs H, in-depth)

Others mentioned the importance of feeling cared for, or loved by, close relatives, for example:

> . . . family . . . just [to] . . . know I'm not completely alone in the world and knowing there's someone who cares about you . . . my brother, his wife, and two daughters and a son, three grandchildren. We are very close, not a big family but a family . . . [I] either visit them or they fetch me out . . . .

The importance of living near supportive others, including neighbours, when health has deteriorated and when people feel vulnerable, was also illustrated by several respondents. Some of their replies are shown below:

> I have a good family, plenty of friends and lots of interests. I have lots of friends that come to wait for me and will take me wherever I want to go – and good neighbours. The man next door takes me shopping and to the doctor's in his car, and his wife does take me shopping if needed. Next door but one the neighbour keeps me company in the evenings.

> Good neighbours – all friendly. Four doors down the man called me to give me broad beans. When I did not put my washing line up he came round to see if there was any problem or I needed help. The lady two doors down does my eye drops three times a week. There is always times I need a doctor, she rings for me. They are all very good to me.

Intergenerational and reciprocal roles can also take on more importance with age – for example, provision of help with practical tasks, shopping, lifts and so on when people are ill or frail, and the role of grandparenting. Respondents said they enjoyed doing things for and with their families, going out with them, as well as seeing them achieve things and progress. Contact with grandchildren, being able to play and go out with them, was frequently mentioned. It was through their grandchildren that people felt able to play a reciprocal role, and felt useful and valued. The reciprocity of the relationship, and the enjoyment of the unconditional love grandchildren could provide, was emphasized in research on grandparenthood by Clarke and Roberts (2004). Similarly, respondents to the QoL survey also said they enjoyed spoiling their grandchildren, and gained pleasure from seeing them happy and feeling loved by them. They also appreciated the practical help, which older grandchildren could provide:

> . . . when the kids come down: they make me die with laughter! [*chuckles*] With all their antics they get up to! It'd be very lonely if our grandchildren were different

. . . They're always on about youngsters today, but . . . I must say that ours are fantastic. They're always here: if we need anything, they're here; when we're going anywhere, they're here; if we want popping up the hospital, or anything, they're here. No problem.

(Mrs V, in-depth)

The quality of my life now is my family – my children and grandchildren. My life surrounds them. I go at weekends, they visit every week. Sometimes I have the younger grandchild staying overnight . . . I can do things with the family. I'm there if they need me. I get them bits for their flat and make them more comfortable. I knit them big jumpers and just look out for them.

My grandchildren. Well I'm noted for activity. I can't keep still. The grandchildren love to come here and go out with me. We like the cinemas, we like the parks, you name it. At least somebody thinks I'm useful . . . The youngest, who is nine, is dyslexic so that can be very awkward. They're too different. They rely on me more – my sons – for hospital appointments, and doctors' appointments, now I've got the time.

Without a reciprocal role, however, some people were afraid of being seen to be a burden by their families, and also referred to their families' own time constraints in providing social contact and support:

Both my daughters' husbands and grandchildren are good to me, but I feel I can't just keep pestering them. I am a little bit independent. They have their lives to live.

And pets were mentioned by some as important, alongside their families, for love (both directions), company and for their pets' 'dependency' on them:

My family – my son, my daughter-in-law and my two grandchildren . . . Oh, and my little cat. I talk to her a lot, she's just like a little child. She doesn't like being left alone, I love her to bits. Now and again I give her a little kiss.

Having good friends, as distinct from neighbours and family, was emphasized by people. They appreciated having company, someone to talk to, the emotional support and close contact which good friends can provide, and, as the following two people illustrated, the fun of going out socially with them:

If I am at home, she (respondent's friend) would come over now and have coffee at 12.30, that kind of thing. We go out to the town on a Saturday and meet her mother for coffee. We go out on a Tuesday night, if we are not dancing we go out to the coffee club and have supper. I'd see most days if I were at home. She's a good friend. She comes over most nights.

(Mrs I, in-depth)

103

Friends isn't it? They take me out for days and we have a social evening once a week. There are six of us and we go round to one another's houses and we play cards . . . We have these clubs for pensioners. I'm in two clubs and they come to fetch us in the buses.

The finding that relatives and neighbours provided practical help, and friends provided emotional support and company, is supported by the literature on social networks and support. The literature also emphasizes the important role of friends and confidants for emotional well-being and for helping to buffer people against the stresses of the gradual losses that can accompany older age (see Bowling 1991, 1994 for review). People with no living relatives or children also compensate with their friendships. As the following woman who had no living close relatives said, the most important thing to her QoL was having friends: 'having friends. I have no family, so friends are terribly important.'

Things that took quality from life

In relation to 'bad' areas of QoL, 12% of respondents mentioned social relationships taking quality away from their lives, although most, 80%, of the in-depth respondents mentioned this (i.e. not having good relationships with friends and relatives, or not having any). Females were more likely than males to talk about poor social relationships in relation to bad QoL: 17%:8% respectively. There were no differences by age or social class. Respondents who were widowed were the group most likely to mention relationships as taking quality away from their lives (i.e. lack of relationships, and missing what they had lost): 24% of those who were widowed, followed by 14% of those who were divorced/separated, 11% of those who were single, 6% of those who were married and none of those who were cohabiting said this. And, as might be expected, respondents who reported feeling lonely 'always', 'often' or 'sometimes' were more likely to mention relationships in terms of bad QoL (44%, 37%, 17% respectively) in comparison with far fewer (7%) of those who said they never felt lonely.

Some of the respondents mentioning this theme also felt responsible for very elderly relatives. They either spoke of the problems caring for ageing relatives in poor health, or having to cope with their deaths, and the organization involved:

Seventeen deaths in the last five years . . . in the extended family, err . . . our responsibilities in that . . . are now over thank goodness – but we had frail relatives in homes or in care of one form or another . . . we have had to do the round of homes, power of attorney, and all the rest of it, and of course that puts a drain on your finances, because you . . . you pay your own fare to go and visit them. Invariably it's a night's accommodation for two, and what do you do when you get there? You don't want to sit in the lounge with other people who are nodding off, err . . . they sit there all week, or all . . . month or whatever since you last saw them, so you put them in the car, and take them out to lunch . . . And then, of course, you'd take him somewhere, maybe walk him to a seat and sit on the prom for an hour, or put him in the wheelchair . . . Err . . . cup of tea, back in the car, back to where they . . . came from. Sort the bills out, and . . . drive home again.

(Mr P, in-depth)

Others reported missing family, friends or a partner who had died for their familiarity, emotional support or love, for doing practical tasks, sharing responsibility and decision-making, or even phone calls:

And my sister-in-law that used to come down every year and used to stay with her brother . . . She died a fortnight, three weeks ago . . . So . . . that hasn't improved me. So I'm getting over that . . . I'm missing all her phone calls on Sundays, I used to phone one week and she use to phone me another and . . . I miss that so I go down to my friends on a Sunday. So I make up for it, somewhere . . . there's some days when I don't speak to a person, I don't speak a word.

(Mrs E, in-depth)

Another recent widow commented that she had no one to socialize with since her husband died, and that her married friends seemed to be avoiding her: 'No hand to hold . . . Socially I am a person *non-gratis*, being seen by other wives as a threat . . . I am pulling myself up, all I want is mature company to help me.' The literature on bereavement has drawn attention to the problem of greater isolation and loneliness among elderly widowed people, and the fact that widowed people can be seen as a threat to friends' spouses (see Bowling and Cartwright 1982).

Social relationships and support, like material resources, tend to be built up over a lifetime. Longitudinal data show that network sizes decrease significantly in older age (Bowling *et al.* 1995a, 1995b; Bowling and Grundy 1998). Although most respondents took part in social activities, they did not tend to see older age as a time for making new close friends, rather that they gained *acquaintances only* from such activities. This led to loss of social support when friends died:

As you get older, all your friends die. How do you live when all your friends are gone? I've lost one em two weeks ago. In an accident down at NR . . . You don't meet any friends when you get older. You can't, you don't go out to meet, and not only that you're old too and friendships takes a long time to . . . I mean I've lost all my friends. I've had another friend that I [*unclear*] she died of cancer at seventy-one. I mean I've lost everybody.

(Mrs P, in-depth)

I had a very good friend GM who died now eight or nine years ago, but we used to talk a lot over problems, but . . . when I lost him, I lost . . . my main supporter from that point of view, 'cause if I wanted to have a chat about something what I wasn't sure about I'd go and see him, and he'd do the same to me, so it was always, it was a mutual thing, but . . . that's the trouble, you lose your confidant, you know . . . the older you get.

(Mr K, in-depth)

Bowling and Cartwright (1982) reported that widow(er)hood, and living at some distance from relatives, can create a dilemma about moving home for older people. This dilemma, and the weighing up of alternatives, was also found among widowed respondents in the QoL survey (see Case 4.1).

Loss of a home has been compared to other forms of bereavement (Hooper and Ineichen 1979), and moving to a new neighbourhood can be bewildering and lonely. However, it should not always be viewed negatively. The widowed respondents who had moved after the death of their spouse in Bowling and Cartwright's (1982) study all said they were glad they had moved when they did. But classic research on older people in general has reported that they prefer not to actually live *with* their children or other relatives (Shanas *et al.* 1968).

This study also indicated that moving in with relatives can be a source of strain, especially when the older person takes on household responsibilities. The following lady moved in with her daughter, hoping to be looked after, but found that she had to take on more domestic responsibilities because of her daughter's poor health:

. . . we sometimes have words and rows in the family. The worry with my daughter – she's not a very good patient, she's got rheumatoid arthritis . . . I do most of the housework. I worry a lot about what's going to happen to us when I get too infirm to do anything. I came here so as not to be on my own, but it's worrying when I came here to be looked after but I do the looking after.

For some respondents, poor social relationships were due to difficulties maintaining contacts or good relationships with their families, either because of geographical distance or family feuds. Some people wanted to see their family more, but spoke of their children and grandchildren being 'too busy' to

---

Case 4.1 Mrs B

Mrs B said her QoL was 'Alright'. She lived by herself in a small village. She said that the good things that affected her QoL were a pleasant home and garden, which she enjoyed maintaining, and a close relationship with one of her neighbours, with whom she went shopping, and good relationships with her children and grandchildren.

> ... they [children] were all up at the weekend 'cause I had a birthday, that was nice 'cause I didn't know D [son] was coming ... And my daughter and her husband were in Tescos, and suddenly a young man came up behind me pushing a trolley, and when I looked round it was D, I had no idea he was coming. So that was lovely ...

However, Mrs B's QoL was negatively affected by living far from her family and not being able to see them regularly. She also missed her deceased husband and being able to go out in his car and do things together. She described how she felt lonely in the evenings and was considering swapping her council house and moving to another town to be nearer to her daughter. However, she was wary of leaving her home and garden, which gave her a lot of pleasure. Her case illustrates the dilemma faced by many older people who are torn between wanting to stay in their own homes and moving nearer their children.

> At the moment, after my family being here – D and my daughter, her husband – and we kept talking and talking of me maybe moving to X, which has given me something to think about. And then you know if it happens I shall get all worried, do I really want to move [*laughs*]? So that's in my mind at the moment, but I was 82 last week, see ... so because of that the common sense tells me it would be good to move really to be near my daughter – if I get much older I might get to the stage where I couldn't even attempt to move ... but because I've got such a nice bungalow and garden it is harder. So you have to weigh that against being lonely.

---

see them. This was sometimes used as a justification to help older people to feel better about not seeing their children and grandchildren regularly:

> I'd like to see my son ... and his children more ... the reason being we think, he just works such long hours ... Our son doesn't get home till about half past seven. We were down there Sunday ... But of course he's got his family, and the boy plays football, and he takes him to football and takes him training on Saturday, and his wife works on Sunday. And so ... his time's taken up.
>
> (Mrs Y, in-depth)

Well, the last time I saw them [her grandchildren] was . . . oh . . . about three and a half years ago. She [her daughter] phones me, now and again, but she's got a busy life, and her husband is a partner in . . . an accountancy firm . . . So I think they've got a lot on in their life, you know: I quite understand, young people, you know. So long as I know she's alright, and the children are fine, and . . . that's all I can hope for, isn't it? Don't expect a lot . . . that's perhaps why I don't get a lot.

(Mrs A5, in-depth)

For others, poor relationships were due to difficulties looking after grand-children:

I have a grandson with learning difficulties, we love him greatly. He comes regularly and we have him a lot because his parents are in business and his quality of life would be bad if we did not have him. At the end of the day I am very tired. He has lack of concentration so he is on a short fuse . . . He does not concentrate on what we tell him to do.

Social roles, social and voluntary activities and hobbies

Most respondents appeared to lead an active and deliberately busy life. Three-quarters of men and women equally said they had been on holiday or on outings in the last 12 months (although this dropped to about two-thirds of men and women aged 75 and over). The majority, 93%, said that in the past month they had engaged in social or leisure activities, either alone or with others, voluntary work, helped to look after someone ill or frail, baby-sat or child-minded. The number of different social activities engaged in was summed; this shows that:

◆ just 7% had engaged in no activities;

◆ 26% participated in 1–2, 34% did 3–4 and

◆ 33% had engaged in 5–12 different social activities over the past month.

In addition, 81% also reported that they had voted in the 2001 election (this did not decline with age, and there were no differences with gender). Political participation is an index of involvement in society, and is similar to figures from other sources (Marmot *et al.* 2003; New Philanthropy Capital 2004).

The important factor in social activities is not just having something to do in retirement and in one's leisure time, but doing something that is enjoyable and important to people. Between 82 and 95% of respondents rated their listed activity as very or quite important to them, except in the case of going to the cinema or theatre, where fewer, 59%, rated it as important. For most (68%) their listed activity was going for a walk, followed by gardening (59%) and

---

Box 4.3 Examples of social activities mentioned

- Walking (68%)
- Gardening (59%)
- Attending clubs or organized groups (42%)
- Going to the library (40%)
- Going to the cinema, theatre etc. (29%)
- Attending place of worship (29%)
- Baby-sitting or child-minding (24%)
- Playing games (physical)/keep fit/sports/swimming (22%)
- Looked after ill/frail person (17%)
- Voluntary work (17%)
- Other activities, including hobbies (10%)
- Attending evening or educational classes (7%)

---

attending a club or local organization (42%). National statistics also show that walking is the most popular physical activity for older people (Walker *et al.* 2001). Box 4.3 summarizes the broad types of activity people engaged in.

The range of social activities included being engaged in helping friends, neighbours or family (e.g. with child care, collecting shopping items), having holidays/weekends away, attending age-related clubs, performing in local arts group/choirs, going to theatre/cinema/concerts/opera, going out for meals, drinks, going on outings/day trips, bingo, gambling on horses, evening and other educational classes, pub quizzes, bridge, going to church and going to the library, undertaking sports/physical activities (swimming, table tennis, cycling, snooker, bowls, dancing, keep fit), gardening and going for walks, including walking the dog. Respondents with dogs commented that walking the dog helped them to meet other people. Respondents undertook a wide range of voluntary work for charities, and for local clubs and committees. Together with the caring and child-minding work they were involved in, the data shows that older people reciprocate and make a large contribution to society in their retirement. Most of the activities that respondents participated in are not exclusively aimed at older members of society but are enjoyed by people of all ages. There were no differences in involvement in activities, or number, by gender, although there was an unexpected small, but significant, difference with age group: 5% of men and women aged under 75 did no activities in the past month in comparison with 10% of those aged 75+.

Participation is social activities varied with social position in society, with those with higher socioeconomic status groups having more social activities than those in lower-status groups. Number of different social activities engaged in over the past month was consistently associated with level of education, social class, income and housing tenure. For example, to take just education, social class and income, 61% of those who had degrees or higher degrees participated in five or more activities in comparison with 23% of those with no formal qualifications. And 48% of those in the highest social classes (professional I and intermediate II) had engaged in more than five different activities in the last month, compared with just 13% of those in the lowest partly skilled and unskilled classes (classes IV and V respectively). This association would be expected as social participation can cost money. Respondents on higher incomes were far more likely to engage in activities than those on lower incomes: 68% of those receiving £19,760 or more per annum had engaged in more than five different social activities in comparison with 25% of those receiving £5200 or less. Again, this is consistent with other research on older people in England (Marmot *et al.* 2003). Chapter 6 shows that self-efficacy was associated with the number of different social activities respondents had undertaken in the past month, suggesting its value as an enabling characteristic. However, the chapter also shows that self-efficacy was also associated with socioeconomic status, suggestive of socioeconomic barriers to it. People in lower socioeconomic groups, then, appear disadvantaged in several directions (e.g. participating less because of the financial costs of social involvement – Crawford 1972 – and also because of lower perceived control over life).

Associations with QoL

Association with QoL ratings   Table 4.1 showed that there was a highly significant association between respondents' social activity score and their self-rated QoL. Thus, those who had participated in the most different social activities in the last month were the most likely to rate their QoL positively.

Finally, as reported earlier, the number of different social activities was also a significant independent predictor of QoL. It was shown in Chapter 3 that adding personal social capital (social networks, support, loneliness and social activities) into the regression model of independent predictors of self-rated QoL increased the change in the adjusted R^2 by 3.1%.

Lay models

Things that gave life quality and things that took quality away from life
Participation in social, leisure and educational activities and also in local

community and voluntary activities was reported to be important to good life quality by 60% of respondents. It was also mentioned by most (80%) of the in-depth interview respondents as giving life quality. This theme was rarely mentioned in relation to bad QoL (by 1% of both survey and in-depth follow-up respondents) (i.e. not having social roles and activities).

Females were slightly more likely than males to say that social activities gave their life quality: 63%:57% respectively. There were no differences with mentioning this theme in terms of age or social class of respondents. And respondents who had a high level of participation in social activities (5–12 or 3–4 activities) were more likely to say social activity gave life quality (69% and 62% respectively) than people with just 1 or 2 activities (50%), or who had no social activities (43%). There were no associations between mentioning (lack of) social activities taking quality *away* from life and respondents' sociodemographic characteristics or social circumstances. However, the 1% of survey respondents who mentioned social activities as a bad area of QoL said this was due to not having any, or the stress or pressure of helping other people.

Social involvement and activity, getting out and keeping 'busy' were frequently mentioned by respondents as coping strategies for preventing loneliness and giving life quality, supporting the notion of a 'busy ethic' in older age (Ekerdt 1986):

> I never sit down, the days just fly by. I think that working voluntary at the hospital is a good eye opener, you get out . . . be thankful it is not me.

> Well, I think being busy really. I'm keen on repairing things and do-it-yourself . . . I play snooker three or four times a week and two evenings I have a couple of pints.

> [QoL] is what you do yourself. You know, if you want to sit and watch television all day, well that's it, perhaps that's your equation of quality of life . . . Mine is to get out and about and do things for myself, or see things that I would like to see or haven't seen, you know . . .
>
> (Mr V, in-depth)

Voluntary work was valued for its reciprocal nature, and people liked to feel both valued and that they were giving something back to society in their retirement. Mr G (Case 4.2) and Mr H (Case 4.3) both described how voluntary work was one way of keeping busy and remaining mentally active after retirement.

Going on holiday or for weekends away was also important for people for relaxation. They also appreciated having a break from their routine responsibilities at home. For example, Mrs O, who had been caring for her ill aunt, and

---

Case 4.2 Mr G

Mr G was widowed and had suffered from a hernia 4 years ago. However, since his wife had passed away 14 years ago, he had undertaken many different types of voluntary work. He had also formed his neighbourhood watch group and served as a volunteer signalman at a preserved railway. Mr G spoke clearly about why doing voluntary work added enjoyment and quality to his life:

> So, helping people . . . does help your own quality of life . . . it gives me such a lot of pleasure to be able to take people and tell, tell them about local history . . . I do slide shows, I've got several different slide shows that I give.

He described it as a way of keeping busy and active:

> I lost my wife fourteen years ago, in fact it was 14 years yesterday since I had to give permission for the [life support] machine to be switched off . . . so I've been on me own . . . ever since. But I think I keep myself busy by doing all these things . . . I mean I'm 77 now but I'm still . . . a volunteer signalman at the [preserved] railway . . . and I think the more active you are, the better quality of life you've got . . . So I do keep myself busy, and I don't believe in sitting . . . watching goggle-box all day long, 'cause I think once you start becoming a couch potato, you soon start, you know, kicking up daisies as I call it . . . I think people . . . do sit down and forget about the quality of life . . . I think the quality of life, you make a lot of it yourself . . . By being active. Once you become inactive I think . . . life's gone . . .

---

often looked after her grandchildren, described how much she enjoyed going away by herself for the first time:

> . . . when you've had a long run looking after people, you feel like a relaxed break, so . . . last year . . . I wanted to get away on my own, and I've never done it in my life . . . and I had a gorgeous time . . . I went to X, with . . . our coach people . . . it really did me good to get away from . . . everyone I knew, and everything that I normally do . . . So I've booked a holiday this year again in August . . . I'm going to Y . . . I think you need to, sometimes, just get that break.

(Mrs O, in-depth)

In addition to mentioning social activities as giving life quality about half (48%) of the respondents mentioned their independent ('solo') activities and amusements – usually undertaken at home, alone – as giving their life quality. These activities included crafts (e.g. woodwork, sewing, knitting

---

Case 4.3 Mr H

Mr H, a widower, said that voluntary work made a large contribution to the quality of his life, and was reciprocal. He was a retired chartered surveyor. Now he was chairman of the board of governors at a local school, he was involved in the local housing society and he served as a magistrate. Rather than pursuing pastimes and worrying about the future, Mr H said he wanted to keep active and give something back to society:

> I want to keep active, I want to contribute to society, and I've been very fortunate in what society's given me, as it were, in successful, professional – and one wants to give something back . . . So that's what I've done.

He also thought that voluntary work was important for retaining mental stimulation. He compared his retirement to his father's:

> I'm very conscious that my father was in the same firm as me before he retired, didn't retire until he was 68, and worked very hard until then. He then cut off every-thing, moved to X on the coast, and he said that's it, finished – and he didn't look after his stocks and shares properly, he wouldn't join the local club which wanted him down there as a treasurer – he said 'No, I've finished' – and within six months he was worrying about dogs' tails [getting shut in doors] and that sort of thing, and mentally he went downhill very, very fast over a couple of years. Although physically he lasted another 12 or 13 years . . . I'm not going to go the same way, I'm going to keep this grey matter ticking. Erm, so having been booted out at 55, I've kept my grey matter hopefully ticking.

---

and restoring antiques), cooking and diet, listening to music/radio, watching TV/videos, reading, mental activities (crosswords, jigsaws, competitions), gardening/tending allotment and watching wildlife (e.g. birds, foxes, squirrels). Some were members of the University of the Third Age. Mention of these independent activities as giving life quality was not associated with marital status, household composition or size, age, sex or social class of respondent.

Some respondents were content with their own company and did not want to join social or other clubs. Some of these people described themselves as shy, while others stated that they were very independent and enjoyed doing things alone, partly because they were used to it:

I mean . . . [I was] a lorry driver . . . You get in your cab in England, and there's nobody with you, and you go away for seven days . . . oh, yes, you can talk to people, but err . . . So I'm quite content with my own company, actually . . . because I know I can't upset myself . . .

I would say . . . I have been brought up to be very independent with all these blessed schools that I went to, and all this . . . adapting myself to this, adapting myself to that, and I enjoy my isolation. If people want to know me or get to know me, they must make the effort. I'm not going to join in this, and join in that . . . and I'm not a regular church-goer or anything like that, if I wanted to go, I'd go, I don't want any vicar's things shoved through the post, because . . . why should he think that I'm Church of England, even? I mean, they do that sort of thing, and that annoys me, because, I'm perfectly capable of making up my own mind . . . I do read a lot, I've read a lot . . . Independent, I think you could call me . . . I'm not somebody who goes for hundreds of these free lunches . . . I'm not that type, I don't think. I've never been . . . been far too independent, and . . . I don't want to lose that independence . . .

(Mr Y, in-depth)

Even when people made an active attempt to pursue their own interests and activities to enhance their QoL, sometimes life events made these difficult to continue, as in the case of Mr D. While he initially pursued his hobbies enthusiastically, realizing they were important in preventing mental and physical deterioration, declining health and caring for others who were ill took its toll (see Case 4.4).

Conclusion

The results reported here on the level of people's social contacts, support and activities were comparable with national data from the British General Household Survey (Coulthard *et al.* 2001; Office for National Statistics 2004). A sizeable minority of people were lonely, and had fairly low levels of support. Vulnerability increased with age, with those over 75 being less likely to have someone who could help them in all the areas of life enquired about.

Social relationships was the most common theme which was identified by survey respondents (81%) as giving life quality '(good' QoL). It was also mentioned by almost all of the in-depth interview respondents as giving life quality. Underlying the value placed on social relationships for the enhancement of QoL was the prevention of loneliness, provision of company and entertainment, the need to feel cared for, and having people to call on for help.

Participation in social, leisure and educational activities and also in local community and voluntary activities was reported to be important to life

Case 4.4 Mr D

Mr D was a retired engineer, aged 80. At baseline, he rated his QoL as being good. He suffered from breathing problems, making it very difficult for him to walk and to do some of the things he wanted to do such as gardening. But Mr D had several hobbies, which he pursued avidly at home. He was a radio enthusiast and he enjoyed using his computer and the internet to download music. Here he spoke of how maintaining interests was important for his QoL. He tried to have an active effect on his life in order to prevent decline.

> R: The great thing is to keep an interest, and, and not to vegetate . . . it's not easy to keep an interest as you get older . . . I know . . . a lot of old people my age that don't . . .
> I: And do you think that's a good thing affecting your quality of life, the radio?
> R: Oh, it is a hobby, it's an interest . . . and that's what [*pause*] stops people vegetating . . . some people let go, I have a personal friend, and he's just let go . . . his life consists of the three basic things, Eating, sleeping, and having his bowels moved. You know – we're going back to infancy, aren't we, if you let that happen, it's something that's got to be guarded against.

But a year later, at his follow-up interview, Mr D's life had changed considerably. Overall, he stated that his QoL had declined as his health was not as good. Mr D's breathing problems were worse and he was suffering from pains in his back and chest. He was waiting to see a specialist for a diagnosis. But he had bought a second-hand electric chair, which had helped his QoL. But since baseline interview, his wife had also been diagnosed with Alzheimer's' disease and he was spending a lot more time caring for her. As she could not walk up the stairs, she was sleeping in the dining room and bathing in the kitchen. He had been refused a stair lift for her by social services. He said that, as a result, he had lost interest in his hobbies.

> I: Are you still doing your hobbies? Last time we spoke you were doing the radio and computer.
> R: That has slowed down, I can't arouse the interest. It takes something new to set me going again. I haven't as much time anyway to spend away from J [his wife] . . . I look after J more.

quality by 60% of respondents ('good'), and a further 48% mentioned the value of their own independent hobbies and interests, which they could engage in on their own. Most of the in-depth interview respondents also mentioned the importance of these social and independent leisure activities to their QoL.

Independent activities, as opposed to those which result in social interaction, have been relatively neglected in the research literature on general well-being and health.

In sum, the survey showed that people who reported having the most social activities, and who had someone they could turn to tended to rate the quality of their lives as better than those who were not in such a favourable position. The in-depth interviews illustrated how social activities, hobbies and relationships can influence QoL. People also emphasized the need to keep busy and active, and some enjoyed the reciprocity that voluntary work could give. It was also illustrated how illness, and the need to help care for close others, can threaten the pursuit of leisure activities and broader social roles, with adverse effects on QoL.

Annex I: summary of sub-themes: social relationships

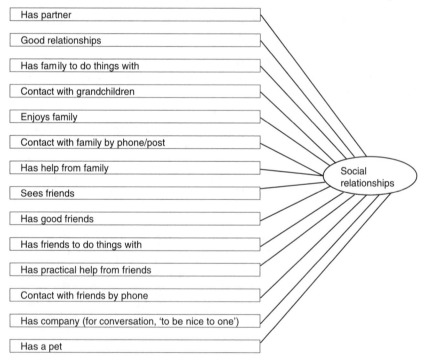

Social roles and activities

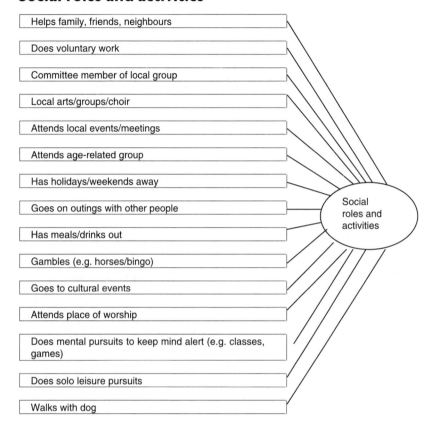

Helps family, friends, neighbours

Does voluntary work

Committee member of local group

Local arts/groups/choir

Attends local events/meetings

Attends age-related group

Has holidays/weekends away

Goes on outings with other people

Has meals/drinks out

Gambles (e.g. horses/bingo)

Goes to cultural events

Attends place of worship

Does mental pursuits to keep mind alert (e.g. classes, games)

Does solo leisure pursuits

Walks with dog

Social roles and activities

5

Health and functioning

You can't buy health, health must be the main source of satisfaction and happiness.

I suppose health's the main thing, cause you've got no quality of life if you haven't got your health, have you?

Despite increases in life expectancy, declining health functioning and restrictions on activities are still common among older people, mainly due to musculoskeletal and cardiovascular disease (Martin *et al.* 1988; Bridgwood *et al.* 2000; Office for National Statistics 2004). British General Household Survey figures suggest that increases in longevity have not coincided with the postponement of ill-health. While levels of serious ill-health and disability are declining, resulting in an increase in life expectancy free of severe disability, more modest levels of health and disability appear to be increasing (Suzman *et al.* 1992; Manton *et al.* 1993, 1995; Dunnell and Dix 2000; Kelly and Baker 2000; Wanless 2002). While 26% of men and women aged 50 to 64 in Britain report a long-term illness or disability, this increases to 74% of people aged 85+ (the rate being higher among women than men at these older ages). Women are also more likely than men to spend more years in poor health. However, it should also be remembered that not all people decline with very old age (see Chapter 10). Bowling *et al.* (1994), in their longitudinal surveys in East London, reported that among people aged 85+ and living at home, some became less mobile, while others improved or stayed the same over a three-year period. Some 'healthy survivor' effects or greater equalization of health risks in very old age, operate in such studies (House *et al.* 1994), but they still highlight the importance of identifying predictors of decline in order to initiate preventive interventions.

As well as having worse health and shorter life expectancy (Machenbach *et al.* 1997), people in lower socioeconomic status (SES) groups, and those exposed to adverse occupational hazards, are more likely to experience disability than others (Adamson *et al.* 2003). Kogevinas *et al.* (1991) also reported that, using housing tenure as an index of SES, council tenants (the lowest

SES group) had poorer survival for cancers of good prognosis than owner-occupiers (highest SES), which might have been partly due to delays in seeking care and/or delays in referral for investigation. Investigators have noted a continuation of the social gradient of morbidity and mortality into older age in population studies (Berkman and Gurland 1998; Avlund *et al.* 2003; Huisman *et al.* 2004; and see Bowling 2004b).

The most frequently reported empirical associations with both well-being and QoL in older age are good health and functional ability. Avoidance of disease and maintenance of physical and cognitive functioning are also, in theory, critical components of active ageing, or successful ageing (Rowe and Kahn 1998). In support of this proposition, health is highly valued by most older people (see Chapter 6). And Bowling's previous research on the important things in life reported that, while older people (aged 65+) gave similar responses to younger adults, their main priority area was their health (Bowling 1995b). As Bond and Corner (2004) suggested, health is perceived to be important to older people's life quality because ill-health is an underlying cause of loss of control, autonomy and independence, and it reminds people of their own mortality.

But, being in poor health is not always equated with poor perceived health or poor QoL. For example, national survey data show that, in 2001, around 1 in 20 men and women in England and Wales considered themselves to be in good health despite reporting a long-term illness which restricted their daily activities. And among those aged 85+ who reported they were in good health, 33% of men and 40% of women reported a long-term illness which restricted their daily activities (Office for National Statistics 2004). Albrecht and Devlieger (1999) explored the QoL of people with disabilities in qualitative interviews. They concluded that a 'disability paradox' existed whereby people with severe disabilities, with apparently poor QoL to an outsider, nevertheless perceived their QoL to be good. Their interviews suggested that this can be explained by respondents (reporting both good and poor QoL) perceiving QoL as dependent on a balance between body, mind and spirit and on maintaining harmony in their relationships. Koch (2000) criticized the concept of a 'disability paradox' on the grounds that self-perceived QoL depends on several factors, not just health and ability. He also pointed to the failure to consider other factors, such as people's coping styles, and their accommodation to changes in their physical status.

Attitudes to health, help-seeking and coping styles may vary by generation, although this has been less frequently investigated by age than by social class. For example, it could be postulated that older people living in the immediate aftermath of the Second World War were likely to have perceived their health as outside their control, and good health as a matter of 'luck'. Minor morbidity was part of life, and doctors were only 'bothered' in the face of major illness. Today, good health, and access to health care, is more likely to be perceived as a human 'right'. But it is largely unknown to what extent today's older people feel this, and to what extent they value their health.

The survey

The questions on functional status (performance of activities, ADL and instrumental activities of daily living, IADL) were based on standard scales (Townsend 1979; Bond and Carstairs 1982; Martin *et al.* 1988), in which respondents rated their ability to perform listed daily tasks on a four-point Likert scale from 'No difficulty' to 'Unable to do alone'. The health status item included was the SF-36 health perceptions item. The standard ONS Omnibus Survey question on self-reported long-standing illness, disability or infirmity was also included.

Health and functioning

As will be shown in Chapter 6, health was valued highly by most respondents, with almost two-thirds agreeing that there were 'few things more important than good health'. Chapter 6 also shows that a sizeable minority were over-optimistic about living to be 100 years of age: 13% of those aged 65<75 and 20% of those who were aged 75+ rated their chances of reaching the age of 100 as higher than other men/women of their age. Most people also rated their health status, and levels of energy, positively. Less than a third said their health was worse than they had expected it to be when they were younger (see Box 5.1). National statistics also show that most older people rate their health positively (Walker *et al.* 2001).

A substantial body of international research has reported the single item measuring perceived health status to be significantly and independently

---

Box 5.1 Perceived health

- ◆ 39% rated their health status, compared with other people the same age, as either 'Excellent' or 'Very good', 34% as 'Good', 21% as 'Fair' and 6% as 'Poor';
- ◆ 77% reported no difficulties with feeling able to get up and do things (energy), although the remainder reported problems;
- ◆ 30% said their health was better than their expectations when they were younger, 42% said it was the same and 28% said it was worse.

---

associated with specific health problems, use of health services, changes in functional status, recovery from episodes of ill-health and mortality (Singer *et al.* 1976; Kaplan and Camacho 1983; Goldstein *et al.* 1984; Schoenfeld *et al.* 1994; Idler and Kasl 1995; Bierman *et al.* 1999; Siegel *et al.* 2003). A review of 27 international studies of self-ratings of health also concluded that the latter is a powerful indicator of mortality (Idler and Benyamini 1997). Hence, perceived health status was analysed in more detail. There were no significant associations with reported health status and age or sex of respondents. Studies in the USA and UK have long reported either no or only slight gender differences with perceived health status among people aged 65 and over (Verbrugge 1985; Bridgwood 2000; Marmot *et al.* 2003). While gender and age differences were found with number or type of diagnosed medical conditions reported, and with level of functional ability (see p. 122–124), the concept of health is more subjective, influenced by individual, social and cultural values and norms (Bryant *et al.* 2001). It cannot be defined in biomedical terms alone, but must be measured by 'the ability of the individual to function in a manner acceptable to himself and to the group of which he is part' (Dubos 1959: 261).

There was an association with perceived health status and socioeconomic status. As would be expected from national datasets (Falaschetti *et al.* 2002; Marmot *et al.* 2003), more of those in the lower social classes IIIm to V, than in the higher social classes I to IIInm, rated their health as just 'Fair' or 'Poor': 31% and 23% respectively. There was also an association between income and health status, with 44% of those whose annual income was over £9360 rating their health as 'Excellent' or 'Very good', compared with 36% of those with incomes below this. Similarly, 42% of those who owned their own homes outright or on a mortgage rated their health as 'Excellent' or 'Very good', compared with 31% of those who rented their accommodation. In addition, respondents with a degree or higher degree were more likely than those with no formal qualifications to rate their health as 'Excellent' or 'Very good': 48% and 37% respectively. Not all the trends with highest education qualification were consistent, indicating the complexity of measuring socioeconomic status among this generation (Grundy and Holt 2001; Bowling 2004b). Other studies have reported on the existence of a clear social gradient with health status, with the lower the social position, the more ill-health and loss of function (Marmot *et al.* 2003).

As would be expected from national data, the most commonly reported physical health problems which respondents said had been diagnosed by a doctor were cardiovascular and arthritic conditions (see Table 5.1). While over a third – 37% (374) – had none of these conditions, and almost a further

Table 5.1 A selection of reported, diagnosed conditions by sex of respondent

Diagnosed condition	Female %	Male %
Other arthritis	22	15**
Heart trouble	18	26***
Osteoarthritis	17	11**
Cancer	10	9±
Osteoporosis	10	2***
Asthma	9	9±
Rheumatoid arthritis	8	6±
Narrowing hardening arteries	7	8±
Bronchitis/emphysema	6	5±
Gout	2	6***
Total	**480**	**518**

**p<0.01, ***p<0.001, ± not significant (chi-square test); some people reported more than one condition so totals do not equal 100%

third had just one (31%) (306), 32% (319) had more than one (between two and six conditions). There were some expected differences by gender and type of health condition reported (Table 5.1), although there were few differences by age. When conditions were summed, however, respondents aged 75 and over were slightly more likely than younger respondents to report having one or more of the listed, diagnosed conditions: 66% and 61% respectively. The significantly higher prevalence of heart disease among men, and of diseases of the musculoskeletal system among women, would be expected, and reflects the long-held observations that the conditions that older men suffer from tend to be life-threatening (e.g. heart conditions), while women suffer from more chronic, disabling conditions (e.g. arthritis) (Sheldon 1948).

More negative self-assessments of health were in response to questions about chronic conditions and physical functioning. For example, 62% reported a long-standing illness, disability or infirmity, and this was frequently said to be limiting (see Box 5.2). This is comparable to national figures (Walker *et al.* 2001).

Consistent with national studies (Bridgwood 2000; Falaschetti *et al.* 2002), there were no significant associations, at bivariate level, with reported long-standing illness and sex, or age when analysed together for both sexes. There were also no associations with long-standing illness and level of educational

---

Box 5.2 Restrictions imposed by reported long-standing illness

- 26% said their long-standing condition limited their ability to care for themselves;
- 42% said their long-standing condition limited their social activities;
- 37% said their long-standing condition limited them in other ways.

---

qualifications or social class (old or new classifications), and differences with income were inconsistent. However, more (70%) of those who rented their accommodation reported a long-standing illness, in comparison with 59% of home owners. The main conditions associated with long-standing illness, and limiting long-standing illness, were cardiovascular diseases, respiratory diseases, hearing and vision problems (the data on health, long-standing illness and functioning have been analysed and reported in more detail by Ayis *et al.* 2003).

In terms of mobility and physical functioning, almost three-quarters (72%) had no difficulty walking 400 yards. However, about a third reported moderate to severe difficulties with the listed everyday tasks, such as housework, shopping and getting out and about. The tasks respondents, particularly women and those aged 75+, had most difficulty with were with: cutting their toenails (37% reported difficulty); shopping and carrying heavy bags (44%); and doing heavy housework (41%).

Responses to 15 listed self-care activities and instrumental activities of daily living (ADL and IADL respectively) were summed to form a score of activities of daily living. The items included were listed in Chapter 2. Just over a fifth of respondents had severe difficulties overall, although at the other end of the spectrum about a third had no difficulties (see Box 5.3).

And again, as would be expected, women were more likely than men to score as having more severe difficulties with ADL or IADL (score of 10–45): 25% and 17% respectively; and people aged 75+ were more likely to score as having

---

Box 5.3 Difficulties with ADL and IADL

- 32% scored as having no difficulties with activities at all (score of 0);
- 33% had slight difficulties overall (1–4);
- 13% had moderate difficulties (5–9);
- 22% had more severe difficulties (10–45).

---

more severe difficulties than younger respondents: 31% and 15% respectively. These difficulties are consistent with the greater prevalence of diseases of the musculoskeletal system among women, and the greater number of all conditions suffered from with increasing older age (see p. 122).

Consistent with other studies, there were significant associations between poor functioning and lower socioeconomic status (Kaplan *et al.* 1993; Seeman *et al.* 1994). Those in the highest occupational (new social class) categories of 'Employers and managers in large organizations' and 'Higher professionals' were less likely to have severe difficulties with ADL or IADL (3%) than those in lower categories of semi-routine and routine occupations (12%). (Although there was a trend with old social class coding also, this did not achieve significance, again indicating the difficulties of using this classification with retired people.) But just 2% of those who had a degree, or higher degree, had severe difficulties with ADL or IADL, in comparison with more, 11%, of those with no formal qualifications. Respondents who rented their homes were also more likely than home owners to have more severe difficulties: 37% and 16% respectively. Finally, those whose annual income was below £9360 were more likely than those with higher incomes to have more severe difficulties with activities: 25% and 15% respectively. Marmot *et al.* (2003) also reported a disability gap between social classes, and argued that it was equivalent to the gap between age groups of ten or more years apart. Chapter 6 reports that high self-efficacy was associated with higher perceived health status and better functioning, suggesting that psychological outlook influences people's perceptions, coping strategies and may have health benefits. However, as higher self-efficacy was also associated with higher socioeconomic status, people in the lower socioeconomic groups are doubly disadvantaged.

Despite functional difficulties, just 10% of respondents were currently receiving help from social services in relation to these, although 27% received chiropody services (provided by health or social services). However, over a quarter of respondents (27%) were able to name practical things that would make their lives easier or better (e.g. having a downstairs toilet).

Associations with QoL

Associations with QoL ratings

Respondents with better perceived health status, with the fewest difficulties with mobility and activities of daily living (both ADL and IADL), and who had no restrictions on their lives due to long-standing illness, were far more likely than others to rate their QoL positively (see Table 5.2).

124

Table 5.2 Respondents' health and functioning characteristics by QoL rating (row %)

Health and functioning characteristics	QoL rating (row %)	
	So good it could not be better/ very good/good	Alright/bad/very bad/so bad it could not be worse
ADL item (1 recoded to 0): able to walk at least 400 yards (n = 992)		
No difficulty (0)	89	11***
Some difficulty (1)	71	29
Can do with aid (2)	74	26
Unable alone (3)	45	55
ADL score ('ADLTOT') (n = 981)		
0 (no difficulties)	91	9***
1–4	87	13
5–9	80	20
10–18	66	34
19–45 (severe difficulties)	55	45
Reported long-standing illness (n = 997)		
Yes	78	22***
No	87	13
Long-standing illness limits participation in social activities (n = 617)		
Yes	66	34***
No	88	12
Long-standing illness limits ability to care for self (n = 616)		
Yes	60	40***
No	85	15
Health compared with other people same age (n = 991)		
Excellent	91	9***
Very good	93	7
Good	85	15
Fair	67	33
Poor	46	54

*** $p < 0.001$ (chi-square test)

As will be shown in Chapter 6, respondents who reported better health status in comparison with their own expectations for themselves were most likely to report their QoL as 'Very good'. Health values, however, were not significantly associated with QoL ratings, although they were useful in indicating the importance of health to most people.

On the other hand, a sizeable proportion of people with severe problems with functional ability still rated their QoL as 'good' in some degree (see Table 5.2), supporting the notion that QoL is made up of factors other than health. It is also possible that dispositional optimism may be operating here, facilitating people's coping behaviour (see Chapter 6), or a strong sense of self-efficacy may help people to adopt a 'can do' approach to life in the face of adversity (Albrecht and Devlieger 1999).

Certainly, in this study, respondents who had moderate to severe difficulties with their everyday activities, and who rated their QoL as good, were more likely than respondents with similar difficulties, but who rated their lives as not good, to have high self-efficacy scores of <13: 59%:37% respectively. In particular, they were more likely than respondents with similar difficulties, but who rated their lives as not good, to feel they had 'A lot' of control over their lives (as opposed to 'Some', 'A little' or 'None at all'): 42%:26% respectively.

Finally, the importance of health and functioning as an independent predictor of perceived QoL was confirmed in the regression modelling. It was reported in Chapter 3 that indicators of health and functioning (ADL score, self-reported health status, reported long-standing illness) independently explained 5.4% of the variance in people's overall QoL ratings.

Lay models

Things that gave life quality

The importance of having and retaining good health for a 'good' QoL was mentioned by 44% of respondents. It was also mentioned by the majority (85%) of the in-depth interview respondents (see Annex I for summary of the sub-themes). And indeed, well over half of all respondents valued their health (see Chapter 6). QoL ratings were consistently associated with having good health and functioning. Those who rated their health as 'Excellent' for their age were more likely than respondents who rated their health less well to mention that health gave their life quality. For example, 59% who rated their health as 'Excellent' mentioned that health gave quality to life, in comparison with 24% of those who rated it as 'Poor'.

Respondents with no difficulties performing ADL were also more likely than those with slight difficulty (score of 1–9), and those with more severe difficulties (score of 10–45) to mention that health gives life quality: 54%:47%:23% respectively. And those who did not report a long-standing illness were more likely to state that health gives life quality: 53% compared with 38% who reported such an illness. There was no association with sex or social class but, probably in reflection of their better health, people aged under 75 were more likely than older respondents to mention that good health and functioning gave quality to their lives: 47% and 39% respectively.

Descartes ([1637] 1953) stated that health is the highest good and contributes to a person's ability to continue in their social roles. And health was reported to be the most commonly nominated important area of life by people aged 65 and over (Bowling 1995b, 1996). Echoing the importance attributed to health in previous studies, having health was highly valued by respondents to the QoL survey as central to their QoL. And as one person summed up: 'You can't buy health, health must be the main source of satisfaction and happiness.' Health was valued for giving quality to life because it was seen as an essential ingredient of retaining independence, being able to do what people wanted and being able to continue driving so they could get out and about. For example, some said:

> Having my health and having a reasonable standard of living. Well they both give you the freedom to do what you want. You are not dependent on anyone . . . I suppose health's the main thing, 'cause you've got no quality of life if you haven't got your health, have you?
>
> (Mrs R, in-depth interview)

> I think that number one is having good health . . . Because without that you are restricted . . . I mean the other things follow on, like being able to go to the gym which I have just done, swim, we play bridge a lot . . .
>
> (Mrs A3, in-depth interview)

In some cases, people prioritized their health because of their negative health events in the past. This is illustrated by the following respondent with a life-threatening condition, who made downward comparisons with others, as well as herself in the past, and thus regarded herself as 'blessed':

> I have just had a pacemaker fitted, and therefore I have been given an extension of my life and therefore there must be a purpose for me, and I use every opportunity to speak to people. I am grateful for a good night's rest and that I can get up in the morning, hear the birds, see the flowers and that I can see. My blessings are that I

can do many things that other people cannot do . . . Many people cannot see, walk or enjoy life so my blessings are many.

Others expressed relief that they were still alive or that they were still living in their own homes, able to do what they wanted to do, which was also linked by them to staying in their own homes. Residential care and nursing homes were seen as stigmatizing and leading to a poor QoL, based on increased dependency and loss of freedom. A dread of moving into residential care was frequently voiced:

> I am still here, I am still in my own home . . . A friend comes in to wash me and I get help from others which means I can keep on living in my own home. I can get about in the house, and I read a bit and watch telly. It's nice here in the summer and I feed the birds. Well, I'm still breathing – just. Just as long as I can stay in my own home.

Coping ability in relation to health was mentioned here in a positive sense. People with health problems referred to making 'the best of things', 'being able to do things despite health problems' and the importance of being able to 'keep going'. For example, Mrs A had cancer, she was also widowed and living far away from relatives. She stated that she thought acceptance of ill-health was her key to successful coping:

> I remember once Dr S said I don't know what you're doing Mrs A but you're doing it right, but I think that was acceptance of what was wrong with me, and trying to make the best and get on with it . . . and carry on as normal . . . I couldn't make an invalid of myself, when you live on your own you've got to do all your jobs and that, no family there, I mean I carried on then as I do now . . . I think acceptance and contentment . . . that's my simple philosophy . . . but I've lived by it . . . and I've got where I am [*laughs*].

A few respondents coped with declining health by making downward comparisons in relation to health, comparing themselves to other people who were worse off, including to their parents' poorer health in the past. They appeared to employ downward social comparisons to help them cope with their problems and maintain their morale or self-esteem. Some people in good health also used this strategy to enhance their feelings of being 'lucky', indicating that health was perceived as due to 'chance' rather than within one's control: 'Seeing other people who are not well makes me feel lucky that I still have good health.'

Things that took quality away from life

Not having good health was emphasized by 50% of respondents in relation to 'bad' QoL, and 83% of in-depth respondents also mentioned this. There was a consistent trend with mentioning poor health as taking quality away from life and health status. For example, 71% of those who rated their health as 'Poor' mentioned this, in comparison with 32% of those who rated their health as 'Excellent'.

As would be expected, those who had more severe difficulties with ADL (score of 10–45) were more likely than those with slight or no difficulties to mention that loss of health took quality from life: 75% in comparison with 49% of those with lesser difficulties and 31% of those with no difficulties mentioned this. And respondents who reported having a long-standing illness, disability or infirmity (61%) were more likely to mention this theme than those who did not report a long-standing condition (29%).

There were no associations with sex or social class of respondents and this theme, although there was an association with age, in reflection of the greater frailty of older respondents: 53% (200) of those aged 75+ mentioned poor health and functioning as taking quality from their lives, in comparison with 46% of younger respondents.

A few respondents made comments concerning the lack of effective medical treatment for their condition, or their fear of planned treatment. For example, the following man was facing a second heart operation, and was afraid, but said he had no option as his condition was life-threatening: 'Not wanting to go through with a second heart operation, which I need because of a leaking valve.' But most of the negative effects of poor health which people mentioned were about 'not being fit enough' to do what they wanted to, being unable to go out and being unable to participate in specific social and leisure and other activities due to ill-health (e.g. sports, playing with grandchildren, walking, hobbies, unable to continue with voluntary work), and being unable to look after themselves or their home (e.g. bathing, housework, shopping, gardening). As would be expected, different conditions had different types of effect on activities. For example, difficulty with hearing led to problems conversing on the telephone, and some respondents said they could no longer listen to the radio or go to concerts. And as one frail woman summed up: 'Well, quality of life . . . the only thing that'd really do me the most benefit is . . . my health better . . . I was always very active, and stuff . . . You can't go . . . because your body's not going with you . . . so, it's a vicious circle, isn't it?' (Mrs A1, in-depth).

And poor health could have multiple adverse effects on QoL. For example, Mrs D's poor health adversely affected her ability to drive and go out independently, and her social activities, although she had tried to compensate and find replacement activities (see Case 5.1). Chapter 1 described psychological theories which emphasized the need to employ compensatory strategies when

Case 5.1 Mrs D

Mrs D was 67 years old at her baseline interview and felt that she had a poor QoL. She had been in an accident eight years before she was interviewed, and she suffered from arthritis in both hip joints. She said that being in poor health detracted from her QoL in several ways. She could no longer drive, and was dependent on her husband for lifts if she wanted to go out, and she found it physically difficult to play with her grandchildren when they came to visit. Mrs D's poor health also meant that she had stopped many of her social activities. But she still looked after her grandson every day while her daughter was at work. Sometimes she had difficulties coping with this and felt that she did not have enough time for herself:

> So my husband and I are left to look after him 90% of the time . . . my daughter works shifts . . . yeah, it's weekends, mornings, take him to school, pick him up, and so he keeps me occupied . . . I've been doing it for seven years. It is getting a bit . . . I used to teach him to cook and garden, he used to put little seeds in pots and things . . . I'd take a seat out to the garden, and he won't do it now, but now he's getting older, he wants to play football, goes mad on his scooter – I can't keep up with him now, so it's getting a bit of a problem . . . if she's working nights he sleeps here . . . And then some nights she finishes at ten, so we take him home, put him to bed and – it's always busy-busy . . . It's just that you can't do the things that you want to do, you know.

Despite these adverse circumstances, Mrs D was still positive during the interview. Her grandson had been born a year after her accident and she was grateful for the opportunity to look after him at this point in her life. Similarly, she found it physically difficult to play with her other grandchildren when they visited, while still enjoying their company:

> R: . . . it's hard work, cause they want to play all the time and of course you can't, so we play cards – we play games that I can sit down to do.
> I: Do you think that affects your quality of life?
> R: I think it helps – it helps you to forget, you know . . . the pain that you're in . . . So we sit and play and bake gingerbread men, and make trifles and things like that . . . it's hard work, it's very painful, but I enjoy it . . . I wouldn't give it up.

Throughout the interview, Mrs D also made several references to coping with poor health and adjusting her life by trying to replace activities she couldn't do with ones she could manage, thus demonstrating how she coped using compensation:

Well it's [the accident] changed it [my QoL] completely. I was outgoing, and I went dancing, and, and, oh, I did everything, flower arranging and night school and walking [*inaudible*] walking and cycling, and it just stopped . . . So now I'm trying to find things that I can do to spend time . . . I had arthritis in one hip which they'd only just found out [about] and it's gone into this one now, so I used to go and play cards while sitting for a long period, but I've stopped playing cards [for long periods] now. I'm knitting instead [*laughs*].

During the year between baseline and follow-up interview, Mrs D's QoL rating had worsened. Her health had worsened, she felt depressed by this, and her relationship with her husband, already strained by her illness and dependency on him, had declined. Linked to her unhappiness with her marriage was the fact that her friends were moving away, so that her own social network had broken down.

facing the dynamic between challenges and depleting reserves for successful ageing (Baltes and Baltes 1990a, 1990b).

Loss of family and friends through death can have a major impact on psychological well-being, physical and mental health. Bereavement can lead to symptoms of nervousness and depression, sleeplessness, loss of appetite, headaches and other somatic problems may be exacerbated by the stress (Bowling and Cartwright 1982). Experience of the process of dying can also be traumatic and can remind people not just of their own ageing and inevitable mortality, but also of earlier, painful losses (e.g. the death of spouse). This is illustrated vividly by Mrs J (see Case 5.2).

And as the next examples illustrate, deteriorating health and consequent social handicaps were reported to have led to depression by other respondents, and to fears for the future, especially when they lived alone or faced cumulative losses:

The end cannot come too soon I suppose . . . I have loads of pain, I'm lonely, unhappy and depressed. I would not care if my next angina attack was my last. I cry every day because I miss my husband so much. I no longer have any social life. Our friends seem to avoid me. I am a lone woman among couples. I have angina which prevents me from doing lots of things – I can no longer go to town shopping.

I think when you live on your own and you're single you worry about what might happen to you if you get ill. If you have your health you can stay in your own

Case 5.2 Mrs J

Mrs J was aged 73 and had been widowed twice. She rated her QoL as 'Very good' at her baseline QoL survey, although she had become depressed after being burgled while she was at home. By the time of her in-depth follow-up interview, Mrs J reported a decline in her QoL. Having lost her sister and two friends suddenly, she had become anxious and depressed:

I: Could we start by talking about anything that has changed in the last year?
R: My sister has died. And ... I've lost two good friends actually, which caused me to have another breakdown or whatever you want to call it – depression, anxiety – that sort of thing ... After those three [deaths] ... So they put me on ... an anti-depressant and I'm still on it.

Mrs J worried about her own deteriorating health, and was afraid of needing hospital treatment because of the poor or ineffective care received by her friends and her sister who had died:

It started actually on 1 November last year. She was my neighbour where I lived before. She fell and broke her hip and she was in hospital and she died on 28 March so she was in hospital quite a long time. I used to go and visit her and I found that terribly depressing because she was in a ward with a lot of very elderly people and she was so unhappy there. That was half the trouble there. She had about three bouts of gastroenteritis while she was in there. She had pneumonia, which she died from in the end. She had an infection in her hip and all sorts of things ... But she got over the actual operation very well and they wouldn't send her out because she had no one to look after her and so they kept her in, but in doing so she caught all these other infections and she died in the end. That really upset me. The other friend I'd known for years too ... he came with his wife for a meal in December and he had been in hospital, the same hospital for nine weeks with some heart problem and they really did nothing apart from change his tablets all the time. And eventually they discharged him and about three weeks after the discharge I invited them for a meal and he wasn't too bad. He did go to sleep after the meal but he ate well and then next day his wife phoned to say that he'd died in the night. I was awfully worried. But he'd had another heart attack. So that was a terrific shock to the system really ... yes ... that was a terrific shock to me ... And then in April my sister died very suddenly ... She'd been to X [on a long-distance flight]. And suddenly, she was playing golf ... when she suddenly became very breathless on the course and just collapsed ... So they took her to M. Hospital. They examined her thoroughly, gave her [an] ECG and said she'd got a chest infection. They kept her there for a few hours but not overnight and they just gave her antibiotics and an inhaler so she went home and they told her to see her GP the next day which she did and she agreed that it was a chest infection and just to carry on as they told her at the hospital. She had no sign of a ... She didn't cough, no pain, she was just breathless. And she was all right when she was sitting down but as soon as she got up and walked around she couldn't breathe so she saw the doctor again and I think they told her to come back in ten days time. But I think she should have gone back before ... My other sister and I visited her on the Sunday. She'd invited us to tea but she couldn't get up and get the tea or anything. We had to do everything. We both thought that she looked very bad so we said you must go to the doctor again and she went back and she said to her well, you know you don't get over these chest infections – you're 78 – at your age very quickly, so come and see me in ten days' time. And she died. Got out of bed on Wednesday and dropped dead. She just couldn't breathe. Then it was discovered that it was a deep vein thrombosis. That was a terrific shock. I knew that she was ill and she was breathless but she'd rung me up on the Monday after she'd seen the doctor and said good we can go on holiday. And the next phone call I had was from her husband on the Wednesday morning saying that she'd died at 9.20 that morning. That was a major shock really and I just went to pieces, I suppose.

This death also led to Mrs J remembering her husbands' deaths more vividly:

My first husband had a pulmonary embolism and as soon as they knew what it was he was in hospital and he [was put] on warfarin or something like that. He got over it but it did leave him with permanent high blood pressure. Of course he died from a heart attack. And it [sister's death] brought it all back. And also her husband that's ... left, he's 81 and is very dependent on me ... It was really terrible just after she died. She had a really good friend who doesn't live too far from me and she used to take me over. We had to do everything, we had to arrange the funeral. That was very traumatic as we were there soon after she died, he [sister's husband] didn't want her to be taken out of the bungalow. He was very upset so my eldest sister and I had to go see them and it brought my two husbands' deaths [back]. It sort of brings everything back ...

Having finally discontinued the anti-depressants a month before her sister passed away, she had started taking them again.

house, it's free, but you do worry about what can happen when you get older. I have friends . . . but I have no family, and they [friends] are the same age, so you couldn't expect to get help there – all getting old together.

The issue of (threats to) independence emerged, and respondents with worsening health disliked greatly their dependence on other people. For example:

First of all I've got impaired sight which is a great drawback and I suppose if I could see life would be a lot different. I'm not independent, that's been taken away from me. I like helping people but I don't like people helping me. I'm very independent and when that's taken away that makes life a misery.

Illness, health generally – the worry that you might not be able to do what you have been doing and what's going to happen next . . . The things I can't do now. I used to play tennis until five years ago . . . If my eyes go I shall lose my independence. I should hate to be dependent on somebody else.

Conclusion

While most people rated their health positively, and had no or few difficulties with mobility, almost four people in ten did have difficulties with tasks such as heavy housework and shopping, and cutting their toenails. Difficulties with ADL and IADL were associated with socioeconomic status: the lower people's socioeconomic status the worse their functioning.

The importance of having and retaining good health for a 'good' QoL was mentioned by 44% of respondents. It was also mentioned by the majority of people at their in-depth interviews. This was generally because health was seen as essential to retaining their independence, being able to do what they wanted to, or continue driving (which also gave them independence). Also, there were consistent associations between mentioning poor health as taking quality away from life and poorer health status, indicating that people valued what they had lost. Among the main dislikes of these respondents were not being able to do what they wanted to and dependency on others. It was also illustrated how ill-health could have multiple adverse effects on other areas of life.

However, respondents also mentioned a range of coping skills which helped them to cope with ill-health. People with health problems referred to making 'the best of things', 'being able to do things despite health problems' and the importance of being able to 'keep going'. Self-efficacy (feeling in control) was associated with perceiving QoL to be good even when faced with poor physical functioning. And in support of the importance of this characteristic, it is reported in Chapter 6 that high levels of self-efficacy were associated with better mental and physical health, suggesting that psychological outlook influences people's perceptions and coping strategies, and may have important health benefits.

These results indicate that policy attention needs to focus on enhancing people's psychological resources, as well as ensuring their access to appropriate health services in order to maintain their health and independence. However, as Chapter 6 also shows, higher levels of psychological resources were also associated with social class. Thus people in higher status groups are more likely to have better functioning and more psychological resources. Marmot *et al.* (2003) argued that being lower in the social hierarchy is equivalent to more rapid ageing. It appears that this also has knock-on effects on people's QoL.

Annex I: summary of sub-themes: health

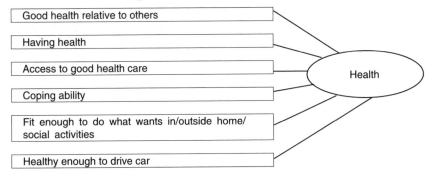

6

Psychological outlook

Quality of life is what you make it, you can't buy it, or inherit it, or anything like that, you know. So . . . as I say, it's what you make it.

[QoL] is what you do yourself . . . Mine is to get out and about and do things for myself, or see things that I would like to see or haven't seen, you know . . . I don't expect to sit back and expect quality of life to come through the door.

. . . and . . . things don't usually work out as bad as . . . pessimists think – so there's no point being miserable if there's no need to be . . . I suppose I certainly intend to enjoy life as long as I can.

. . . I mean, when you're getting older, and you've got these . . . ailments . . . you've just got to accept them and learn to live with them.

In this chapter the focus is on psychological outlook, including health, in relation to QoL. The breadth of this topic is wide and includes psychological health and morbidity (e.g. symptoms of anxiety and depression), optimism-pessimism, self-efficacy (perceived mastery and control over life), social expectations and comparisons, and selected values and perceptions. It was pointed out in Chapter 1 that there has been an increasing body of literature suggesting that attributes of personality and psychological make-up are important for a person's perceived well-being and QoL in older age. Several psychological variables have been hypothesized as key predictive factors of perceived life quality. These include level of adaptation, self-efficacy (mastery and control), independence and autonomy, morale and self-esteem, social comparisons and expectations of life, optimism-pessimism bias, social values, beliefs, aspirations and social comparison standards, selection, optimization, compensation, positive/effective adaptation and coping strategies (Baltes and Baltes 1990b; Day 1991; Wenger 1992; Lawton 1996). Some of these characteristics are related. The literature on coping also provides evidence that personality characteristics, such as optimism and high perceived self-mastery are related to better coping mechanisms (Pearlin and Schooler 1978; Scheier and Carver 1985).

Most research literature on psychological health and well-being in older age groups relates to psychological morbidity and life satisfaction (see Bowling *et al.* 1991, 1999). Survey questions on happiness, well-being and life satisfaction have become a regular part of national population surveys and market research in the USA and Europe (e.g. the Boots Company's 2002 *Well-being Customer Survey*). High rates of life satisfaction in older age have been reported, although a fifth to a third of people aged 65+ have low life satisfaction (Bowling and Browne 1991; Bowling *et al.* 1991). On the negative side, the most common psychiatric diagnosis among community samples of people aged 65 and over is depression. Prevalence surveys vary, probably due to the use of different measures, but estimates for severe depression in this group, across Europe and the USA, are around 10–13%, increasing to 20–27% if less severe categories are included, with depression being higher among the very elderly (Bowling and Browne 1991; Bowling and Farquhar 1991). Rates of increase, or decline, of both life satisfaction and symptoms of depression with older age have also been reported to vary by gender; and poor physical health and physical functioning have been reported to be the most powerful independent predictors of both life satisfaction and psychological morbidity among older people in Britain, including among the very old (see Bowling 1990; Bowling and Browne 1991; Bowling and Farquhar 1991; Bowling *et al.* 1991).

Consciously or unconsciously, rather than succumb to depressive symptoms, most people accommodate or adjust to deteriorating circumstances, whether in relation to health, socioeconomic or other factors, because they want to feel as good as possible about themselves. The roots of this process of adaptation are in control theory, with response shift as a mediator which aims for homeostasis; thus, internal standards and values change (and hence perceptions of QoL) (Sprangers and Schwartz 1999). There are likely to be other, unknown mediating factors that affect perceptions of life quality which might lead people to accommodate to deteriorating circumstances, and thereby lead to perceptions of a higher QoL (Diener *et al.* 1991; Sprangers and Schwartz 1999). The whole topic is complex, and it is largely unknown which psychological variables mediate, and which influence, perceived life quality. Baltes and Baltes (1990b) emphasized the importance of being able to employ compensatory strategies, 'selective optimization with compensation', when facing the dynamic between challenges in life and depleting reserves (e.g. when facing illness or frailty). For example, when selected activities have to be discarded (e.g. due to ill-health or bereavement), strategies need to be activated in order to find new ones and to maximize the chances of maintaining reserves. There is some supportive evidence that these strategies are associated with higher levels of life satisfaction and QoL (Freund and Baltes 1998).

While in theory it might be expected that these strategies would enhance self-mastery, and hence one's perceived independence, control and autonomy, there are often constraints imposed by the hierarchical social structure of societies. Thus, people in low socioeconomic status groups, with lower levels of control over some main areas of their lives (e.g. finances), have been reported to be more likely than those in higher status groups to experience low self-esteem, self-efficacy and self-mastery (Blacksher 2002). However, Doyal and Gough (1991) argued that there are two basic human needs, health and autonomy, which are absolute, not relative to a particular culture. This approach overlaps with Sen's (1992) focus on capabilities, and it could be argued that the achievement of autonomy or capability is essential for individual freedom. There is also evidence that lack of autonomy, or control over one's life, leads to poor health outcomes (Marmot *et al.* 1997; Hemingway and Marmot 1999). In addition, longitudinal data from people aged 70–79 in the MacArthur studies of successful ageing has shown that beliefs in one's self-efficacy has had a significant impact on functional and cognitive ability (Seeman *et al.* 1996b, 1999).

Relevant to this is positive affect (e.g. optimism, feeling hopeful about the future, self-confidence, enjoyment of life) (see Ostir *et al.* 2004), also widely recognized as having protective benefits against poor health and physical functioning, including reduction of risk of adverse medical events such as stroke and myocardial infarction (Scheier *et al.* 1989; Fitzgerald *et al.* 1993; Segerstrom *et al.* 1998; Ostir *et al.* 2000, 2001a, 2001b, 2004), although research has also been inconsistent. Dwelling on negative thoughts is likely to lead to depressed feelings, while focusing on things that have gone well can promote positive feelings. The theory is also that an optimistic mind assists the body's immune system to fight disease and delay the ageing process. It has been reported to be associated with higher levels of engagement is social activities (Ryff and Singer 1996), better coping abilities in the face of stress (Folkman 1997) and greater perceived control over life (Ryff and Singer 1996). Positive psychologists, reminiscent of positive-thinking movements, in contrast to geneticists (Lykkken and Tellegen 1996), believe that optimism can be learned – that people can learn to see a bottle half-full instead of a bottle half-empty, and that having a happy outlook is a skill which can be cultivated (Seligman 2004).

It is over 2300 years since Aristotle began to ponder on how to live life well, and the quest for happiness is still an increasing preoccupation of the developed world. Happiness, well-being and life satisfaction are believed to be relative concepts, and linked to social expectations and to type of comparisons made of oneself with others. For example, people employ social comparisons with others as a reference level when making their assessments of themselves, and this varies for different people (Brickman and Campbell 1971). And in contrast to well-being, which is a relatively stable characteristic, happiness can fluctuate within short time periods. As was pointed out in Chapter 1, social comparisons are one of several ways in which people cope with the problems they are facing, by constructing and evaluating the gap between desired and achieved reality (Sherif 1936; Hyman 1942; Festinger 1954). They may also act as mediators to the effects of adverse events and circumstances (Heidrich and Ryff 1993b, 1995). It is believed that focusing on the things which makes one less like those who are 'worse off' leads to a better sense of well-being.

One of the main psychological strategies proposed for maintaining well-being and promoting self-mastery and control in the face of the challenges of ageing is the use of self-enhancing social comparisons (e.g. when in poor health) (Ryff 1999). It is believed by some that if people make upward comparisons of themselves and their circumstances with others who are better off, then they are more likely to be unhappy, dissatisfied with their lot and have unmet expectations than people who make downward comparisons of themselves with others who are worse off. When appraising their aspirations, most people choose their level of aspiration as higher than what they have but at an attainable level, and their standards of comparison act as a level against which progress can be measured. In this view, real happiness is achieved if people perceive themselves progressing to this level of aspiration. Such relativist theories provide little information about objective QoL (people's overall circumstances), justified by the fact that levels of satisfaction with the same objective circumstances (e.g. income) vary. In contrast, it was pointed out in Chapter 1, Veenhoven (1991) and others have argued that relativistic theory is incorrect, and that QoL ratings increase with objective improvements in life (e.g. living standards). However, while there is evidence to support both positions, suggestive of a compromise stance; the relativism vs. absolutism debate continues.

The survey

Measures of psychological health and outlook included the 12-item version of the General Health Questionnaire (GHQ-12) (tapping general psychological, non-psychotic, morbidity, mainly anxiety and depression); and items on self-efficacy (Schwarzer 1993), optimism-pessimism (Sheier and Carver 1985), real-unreal optimism-pessimism (Sutton 1998) and health values (Lau *et al.* 1986).

Psychological health and morbidity

The majority of people rated themselves as able to make decisions, able to face up to problems, having self-worth and generally happy (see Box 6.1). The items which indicated problems with psychological health mostly related to concentration, feeling useful, strained, enjoyment of activities and unhappiness/depression. Eight in ten people had no symptoms of psychological morbidity (e.g. anxiety/depression), although this left a fifth who scored as having psychiatric morbidity ('cases'). This is consistent with the prevalence figures given earlier for broader definitions of depression (severe and less severe cases combined).

Respondents with good psychological health (non-cases) were more likely than those with poor psychological health (cases) to make downward social comparisons with people worse off than themselves: 40% made these (having the highest comparison scores of 14+) in comparison with 22% of cases. This is consistent with gap theory which holds that people should make downward

---

Box 6.1 GHQ items indicating no psychological problems (non-cases) with items tapping:

◆ Concentration	76%
◆ Sleep	82%
◆ Feeling useful	80%
◆ Decision-making	87%
◆ Strain	79%
◆ Overcoming difficulties	88%
◆ Able to enjoy activities	76%
◆ Facing up to problems	91%
◆ Unhappy/depressed	80%
◆ Confidence	85%
◆ Self-worth	93%
◆ Happy	91%

Case of psychological morbidity (score of 4+): 20%

---

social comparisons to boost their self-esteem and make themselves feel better about their own situations, thereby boosting their mental health.

Those with good psychological health were also more likely to score best in self-efficacy (score of 5–10 on the scale of 5–23): 29% compared with 12% of those with poor psychological health, which is again consistent with the theory described earlier on psychological resources and QoL. They were also more likely to be optimists (see p. 143). Psychological outlook was reported to be preventive of depression among older adults by Schieman et al. (2002; Schieman and Meersman 2004).

As with physical functioning (see Chapter 5), there was evidence of social inequity in relation to psychological functioning. Those in good psychological health were more likely to be categorized as employers and managers in large organizations, and higher professionals (new social class coding). For example, 84% of these respondents scored as non-cases with the GHQ, in comparison with 70% of those in the lowest category of routine occupations. There were, however, no associations with old social class coding. And 87% of those with a degree or higher degree scored as non-cases, in comparison with 77% of those with no formal qualifications.

Self-mastery and control over life

Almost two-thirds of respondents (61%) scored as 'high' to 'middle high' in self-efficacy overall, almost a quarter (23%) had middle-low scores, 16% had the lowest self-efficacy scores. Box 6.2 shows the items which were included in the self-efficacy scale, and summarizes the results for those scoring high in self-efficacy. While over three-quarters agreed that they tried harder in the face of failure, just over half of respondents expected things to work out the way they wanted them to, and less than half in each case felt that they could make their plans work and did not expect things to go wrong for them. This shows that large percentages of respondents had high self-efficacy, and most of the remainder fell into the middle categories, rather than at the extreme negative ends of the spectrum.

High self-efficacy was associated with higher perceived health status: 32% of those rating their health for their age as 'Excellent' or 'Very good' had the highest self-efficacy scores (of <11) in comparison with 24% of those who rated their health as 'Good' and 18% of those who rated it as 'Fair' or 'Poor'. Those with no problems with ADL (ADL score of 0) were also more likely than those with problems to score highest in self-efficacy: for example, 31% of those with no ADL problems scored highest in self-efficacy compared to

---

Box 6.2 High self-efficacy: 'Strongly agree'/'Agree' responses

- ◆ Tries harder in the face of failure   78%
- ◆ Expects things to work out well   53%
- ◆ Can make certain plans work   47%
- ◆ Does not expect things to go wrong   43%

- ◆ Amount of control over important things in life: A lot   44%
                                                        Some   45%
                                                        Little or none   11%

High, middle high scores for self-efficacy (<13) ('EFFIC'):   61%

16% with the severest problems (ADL score of 19–45). It was reported earlier that high self-efficacy was associated with psychological health (non-case with the GHQ). It is possible that psychological resources influence people's perceptions of their coping abilities and functioning, and may have indirect health benefits.

That self-efficacy was also an enabling characteristic in life is supported by its association with the number of different social activities respondents had undertaken in the past month. There was a consistent trend between scores, with 34% of those with the highest number (5–12) of social activities having the highest self-efficacy score, in comparison with far fewer, 11%, of those with no social activities in the last month. And people who could ask for help and support in all five areas of life questioned about (see Chapter 4) were more likely to have the highest self-efficacy scores than those who had support in less than three areas: 28% compared with 10%.

As would be expected, structural features of society and people's socio-economic position influenced perceived self-efficacy. Scores were significantly associated with all socioeconomic indicators, in the expected directions. People with the highest socioeconomic status – with the highest level of education, the highest incomes, in the highest social classes, and those who were home owners – were advantaged by being more likely to have the highest self-efficacy. Almost half, 45%, of those who had a degree or higher level of education had the highest self-efficacy scores, in comparison with 21% of those with no formal qualifications. Similarly, 42% of those with an annual income of £19,760 or more had the highest self-efficacy, compared with 35% of those with £14,560 but less than £19,760, and far fewer, 23%, of those with less than this. Just under a third, 30%, of those in the higher social classes (I professional to III non-manual) had the highest self-efficacy, compared with just 14% of those in lower social classes (III non-manual to V unskilled). And over a quarter, 27%, of home owners had the highest self-efficacy, compared with 5% of those who rented their accommodation. Finally, 29% of those with access to a car or van in the household had the highest self-efficacy, compared with 19% of those without such access. Macintyre *et al.* (2000) also reported that home ownership was associated with higher self-mastery, and that access to a car was seen by people to be enabling, again leading to enhanced self-efficacy. Hence there are social barriers to enhanced self-efficacy which positive psychology needs to take account of.

Optimism

Previous research has reported that most older people consider themselves to be optimists (see Chapter 1). While seven in ten people in this study said they tended to look on the bright side, just under half tended to expect the best (see Box 6.3). The summed items on optimism showed that, overall, two-thirds were categorized as optimists.

Again, consistent with psychological theory, having an optimistic outlook appeared to protect against psychological morbidity, as people in good psychological health (non-cases with the GHQ) were more likely to have the most positive optimism scores: 69% compared with 51% of those in worse psychological health (the latter may reflect pessimism bias in the cases of depression). There were no trends with socioeconomic status.

Perception of risks to self: realistic and unrealistic optimism-pessimism

Another method of tapping levels of optimism and pessimism, both real and unreal, is to examine realistic and unrealistic estimates of self-risk (Sutton 1998). Respondents were asked whether they estimated their risks, in relation to other men/women (gender matched to sex of respondent) of the same age,

---

Box 6.3 Optimism: 'Strongly agree'/'Agree' responses

- Always look on the bright side   70%
- Expect the best in uncertain times   49%

Optimists on summed scale ('OPTIMIST')   66%

were higher, about the same, or lower in relation to a series of life- and health-related events. In questionnaire design, categories such as 'same as others' or 'no more than usual' are generally regarded by respondents as referring to an average or usual state, and not as high risk categories, although there is some debate about this (Goodchild and Duncan Jones 1985; Goldberg and Williams 1988).

Table 6.1 shows that there was little evidence of unreal pessimism. People appeared to be fairly realistic, on the whole, with the possible exception of their risk of getting some of the health conditions. However, there was a higher degree of unreal optimism in relation to the chances of becoming a centenarian. Most people rated their chances of the listed events as about the same as for others, with the exception of being mugged, where similar proportions rated their chances as lower or the same as others their age. Despite many people voicing concerns about their personal safety (see Chapter 7), substantial proportions considered themselves to be at lower risk of being mugged or burgled.

There were significant associations between higher rated chances of being mugged and lower social class, and between higher rated chances of being

Table 6.1 Respondents' ratings of event happening to them, compared to other men/women their age (row %)

Chances of event happening to them (*n* = 968–989+)	Higher	Same	Lower
Being mugged	9	45	46
Being burgled	8	54	38
Falling and breaking a bone	15	65	20
Being knocked down crossing the road	11	57	32
Getting cancer	7	75	18
Getting heart disease	7	66	27
Losing memory	6	76	18
Becoming housebound	7	68	25
Going into nursing home	4	58	38
Living to be 100	16	57	27

+ The totals for three items were lower than these: heart disease (462), cancer (859) and becoming housebound (841); these reflected the higher numbers of ineligible respondents who were not asked the question as they had already reported these circumstances knocked down crossing the road and lower social class. For example, 65% of those who rated their chances of being mugged as higher were in the lower social classes of IIIm to V, compared with fewer, 49%, of those who rated their chances as the same as others, and 36% of those who rated their chances as lower. And 63% of those who rated their chances of being knocked down as higher than others were in the lower social classes of IIIm to V, in comparison with fewer, 45%, of those who rated their chances to be the same, and 38% of those who rated their chances as lower. These associations are likely to reflect some degree of realism, as they are likely to reflect the increased incidence of such adverse events in the area of residence of people in lower socioeconomic groups (higher density, striving areas, with lower social capital) (Dodd *et al.* 2004; see also www.homeoffice.gov.uk).

Only 15% of respondents thought their chances of falling and breaking a bone were higher than others. In fact, every year in the UK, a third to half of people aged 65 and over have a fall, and half of these will have another fall within a year. Falls are a major cause of disability (e.g. from hip fracture) and the leading cause of mortality (see National Institute of Clinical Excellence 2005). Those who rated their chances of falling to be higher than others were being realistic. About a third (31%) of respondents had actually fallen in the past 12 months, although breaking a bone was uncommon. And 45% of those who rated their chances of falling and breaking a bone as higher than others had actually fallen in the past 12 months, in comparison with fewer, 29%, of those who rated their chances as the same, and 17% of those who rated their chances as lower.

Apart from falling and breaking a bone, the item where a sizeable minority of respondents rated their chances of the event occurring as higher, related to the only positive event in the list: living to be 100 years of age (by 16%). This indicates some degree of unrealistic optimism as less than 1% of people aged 65+ in the UK are aged 100 or more, and the numbers are expected to increase to 1% by 2066 (Office for National Statistics 1999).

People also demonstrated realism in response to the item about entering a nursing home. Just 4% rated their chances as higher, broadly reflecting national data (between ages 65 and 74 the chances of living in long-stay care was 1%, rising to 5% at ages 75–84, and 20% at age 85+) (Laing and Buisson 2004). Just 6% rated their chances of losing their memory as higher than others. This reflects some degree of realism as current figures show that 5% of people aged 65 and over in the UK will develop dementia, although this rises to 20% among people aged over 80 (see www.alzheimers.org.uk).

What is striking from the responses to the health condition events, given that heart disease and cancer are the most common causes of death among older people, is that over a quarter of respondents rated their chances of getting heart disease as lower than that of others the same age, and almost a fifth rated their chances of getting cancer as lower. However, these questions were only asked if respondents had not already reported these conditions (and they may be the 'healthy survivors'). Future follow-up can assess whether these perceptions were due to unrealistic optimism. There were no associations with socio-economic status and ratings of chances for the health-related events, which suggests some degree of unrealistic optimism among people in the lower social status groups, given their known higher mortality risk and worse functioning.

Health values

The two items on health values were based on Likert scale responses to statements about the importance of health to people, and how much they cared about their health. As Box 6.4 shows, health was certainly important to most people. Between 57 and 62% of respondents indicated that they valued their health. There were no associations with socioeconomic status, indicating that health was valued equally by all groups. The salience of health to older people is consistent with the author's previous work on the things that people say are important to them, in which health was reported to be the most commonly nominated area of life by people aged 65+ (Bowling 1995b, 1996). And it was shown in Chapter 5 that having health was highly valued by respondents as central to their QoL.

Social comparisons and expectations in life

Social comparisons are regarded in psychology as positive coping behaviour and are important to well-being in later life. A series of questions was asked about expectations of life and how respondents compared themselves and

---

Box 6.4 Health values

- I care about many things more than my health
  ('Strongly disagree'/'Disagree')   57%

- Few things are more important than good health
  (Strongly agree'/'Agree')   62%

Box 6.5 Social comparisons and expectations

Living conditions and financial situation	%
Has more than expected	42
Same as expected	36
Worst off than expected	22
Feels a lot better off than expected when younger	25
Feels a little better off	28
Neither better nor worse off	19
A lot/little worse off	28
Feels a lot better off than others like self	31
Feels a little better off	11
Neither better nor worse off	43
A lot/a little worse off	15
Life achievements	
Done everything/most things in life they had wanted to	53
Some of the things	38
Done few or none of the things	9
Highest (best) 'GAP' summed score:	37%

their circumstances to others. Between 42 and 53% of respondents felt they were better off than other people like themselves, or than they had expected, in general and when they were younger ('in your 40s'), although between 15 and 28% said they felt worse off (see Box 6.5).

In addition, people were asked about their achievements in comparison with what they had expected for themselves ('Thinking about the things you have done in your life and the things you would like to have done . . .'). Most people said they had done all or some of the things they had wanted to do.

When items were summed, over a third (37%) had the best social comparisons and expectations ('GAP') scores (indicating feelings of being better off, with met expectations overall), and although most other respondents fell into the middle ranges (39%), about a quarter (24%) scored badly. The latter are likely to be a potentially vulnerable group, with unmet expectations, making upward social comparisons and thus creating dissatisfaction. There were no associations with socioeconomic status.

It was reported earlier in this chapter (see p. 140) that psychological health, as measured by the GHQ-12, was associated with gap scores in the expected direction. Gap score was also associated with income, with slightly more respondents who had less than £9360 per annum scoring worst (score of 5–10) than those with higher incomes (20%:16% respectively). Inevitably, those on the lowest incomes may find downward comparisons more difficult and may make the most negative social comparisons. Positive psychology has ignored these social differences.

Associations with QoL

Associations with QoL ratings

Table 6.2 summarizes dichotomized QoL ratings by selected psychological variables. The trends with QoL were in the expected directions. Those who were optimistic, with more positive self-efficacy, no psychological morbidity (non-cases with the GHQ-12), and those who rated themselves at lower risk of negative life and negative health events were more likely to rate their quality of lives highest. There were no associations with health values. People whose financial circumstances and health were better than they had expected them to be, and who thought their circumstances were better than other people's (of the same age) were more likely to rate their QoL positively. This indicates the importance of making downward social comparisons for one's well-being and self-esteem (i.e. to make oneself feel better off). These associations were consistent when analysed by the full range of QoL ratings (undichotomized), and also with the individual items that made up each of the summed scales shown.

Finally, it was reported in Chapter 3 that the main *independent predictors* of self-rated global QoL were: social comparisons and expectations (adjusted R^2: 6.4%) and personality and psychological variables (optimism-pessimism retained statistical significance within this model). Adding the latter to the model increased the amount of explained variation to 14.6% and these variables explained most of the variance in QoL ratings (increasing the change in the adjusted R^2 by 8.2%). These findings support psychological theories of enhanced QoL in older age.

Lay models

Things that gave QoL

Psychological outlook and well-being was mentioned by 38% of survey respondents in relation to 'good' QoL. It was also mentioned by almost all

148

Table 6.2 Respondents' psychological characteristics by QoL rating (row %)

	QoL rating (row %)	
Psychological characteristics:	So good it could not be better/very good/good	Alright/bad/ very bad/so bad it could not be worse
Optimism-pessimism score ('OPTIMIST') (n = 989)		
<6 (optimist)	84	16***
6–7	78	22
8–10 (pessimist)	81	19
Social expectations and comparisons ('GAP') score for finances and standard of living (n = 947)		
5–10 (worse-off compared to expectations/others)	71	29***
11–13	83	19
14–16	88	12
17–20 (better off compared to expectations/others)	93	7
Social expectations and comparisons ('GAPTOTAL') score (includes finances, standard of living and health expectations) (n = 929)		
<11 (worse-off compared to expectations/others)	63	37***
11–13	73	27
14–16	87	33
17–23 (better off compared to expectations/others)	92	8
Health compared with expectations (n = 972)		
Better	89	11***
Same	86	14
Worse	68	32
Health value score (n = 988)		
<4 (values health high)	81	19±
4–5	82	18
6+ (value health low)	83	17
Self-efficacy score ('EFFIC') (n = 983)		
<11 (high in self-efficacy)	89	11***
11–12	86	14
13–14	78	22
15–23 (low in self-efficacy)	69	31

Total psychological outlook score ('EFFICACY') (includes self efficacy, optimist, health values)
(n = 981)

5–10 (high in self-efficacy and positive outlook/values)	88	12**
11–12	88	12
13–14	81	19
15–23 (low in self-efficacy and positive outlook/values	73	27

Perception of risks of adverse life, health and frailty events score ('RISKTOT')+ (n = 359)

<19 (high self-risk)	81	19**
20–22	91	9
23–27 (lower self-risk)	85	15

Perception of risks of adverse life events (minus health, frailty events) ('RISKASAC)++ (n = 976)

<8 (high self-risk)	69	31***
8	85	15
9–10	86	14
11–12 (low self-risk)	82	18

Perception of risks of adverse health and frailty events ('RISKHEAL')+++ (n = 360)

5–9 (high)	74	26**
10	85	15
11–13	86	14
14–15 (low risk)	95	5

Perception of risks of adverse frailty events ('RISKFRAI')++++ (n = 828)

2–3 (high)	66	34***
4	88	12
5	86	14
6 (low risk)	90	10

Psychological morbidity: GHQ-12 score ('GHQCASER') (n = 990)

1–3 (non-case)	86	14***
4–12 (case)	68	32

+ Self-assessed chances of being mugged, burgled, falling and breaking a bone, knocked down while crossing the road plus getting heart disease (where condition not reported), cancer (where condition not reported), losing memory, going into nursing home, becoming housebound (where condition not reported)
++ Self-assessed chances of being mugged, burgled, falling and breaking a bone, knocked down while crossing the road
+++ Self-assessed chances of getting cancer (where condition not reported), heart disease (where condition not reported), losing memory, housebound (where condition not reported), going into nursing home
++++ Self-assessed chances of becoming housebound (where condition not reported), going into nursing home
**p<0.01, ***p<0.001, ± not statistically significant (chi-square test)

(96%) of the in-depth interview respondents as giving life quality (see Annex I for summaries of the sub-themes). There were no differences with mentioning this theme as giving life quality and age, sex or social class of respondent. There were also no associations with having an optimistic or pessimistic disposition and mentioning this theme. However, respondents with no psychological morbidity (GHQ-12, mainly anxiety/depression) were slightly less likely than those who scored as such cases to mention psychological outlook and well-being as giving life quality: 31% and 39% respectively. The respondents who mentioned this theme often referred to the importance of being realistic, acceptance of unchangeable circumstances, taking each day as it comes, not worrying about the future and 'making the best of things': '. . . there's not a lot you can do about that [poor health with age], as I said you've got to take one day at a time, and live that way. One day at a time . . . that's what we do . . .'.

But along with acceptance, they also emphasized the importance of having a positive mental outlook in influencing the quality of their lives, specifically having a positive or optimistic disposition (being a happy/satisfied/enthusiastic/content person), having good memories of the past (job, family, achievements) and being able to look forward to things. These strategies were said to help some people cope when overcoming bereavement and poor health. For examples see Box 6.6 and Case 6.1.

Box 6.6. Psychological coping strategies

I suppose I'm a bit of an optimist, in a way – and I think my husband's probably a pessimist [*laughs*] . . . I enjoy life, put it that way. I think there's no point in living if you're not enjoying yourself, so you might as well enjoy yourself, and . . . things don't usually work out as bad as . . . pessimists think – so there's no point being miserable if there's no need to be . . . I suppose I certainly intend to enjoy life as long as I can . . .

(Mrs C, in-depth)

I'm an optimistic person, I look on the bright side. It's no good looking at what might happen, because people worry themselves into the grave thinking if, you know, I'd better not go outside because I might fall over. That's silly. I think the one thing that when you get old . . . you've really got to think hard about is that when you go out . . . you think 'I mustn't fall over

---

because if I break a leg I can't get around anywhere'. So you rather, as it were, tread gingerly, a little bit. Because the one thing that'll put you out of action is if you break a leg. If you break an arm you can still walk around, you know.

(Mr G, in-depth)

I think acceptance – I've found when I've had, like when my first husband was killed in a road accident, and my second husband, he sat and died suddenly . . . you've got to accept that these things have happened, and you've got to move on. I think so anyway . . . I mean there's some people [*inaudible*] oh, she'll never get over that, well you never do get over it but if you can accept it you can start taking the steps, you've got to . . . life's got to go on, hasn't it? I think acceptance and contentment, they're the sort of things . . . That's my simple philosophy . . . But I've lived by it . . . and I've got where I am [laughs].

(Mrs F, in-depth)

I: What makes you the most happy at the moment?
R: I don't know . . . I'm very even-tempered – I keep equilibrium. There's nothing that exhilarates or depresses me. I don't sit here thinking 'Oh I'm going to the theatre tonight.' I don't sit here thinking or anticipating things – for example, the theatre – I just get there and enjoy it . . . or not.

(Mr Y, in-depth)

I'm a content lady . . . 'cos I've got my home and my garden . . . I'm satisfied . . . As a family we never had a lot, my dad died when we were little tots, so we've never been a lot of money in the family, so I've never been one that's brought up to want, want, want, you know, I mean I've got neighbours and friends, says they've got to have this, they've got to have that . . . For me there's a lot of things I would like, but I can't afford them, so I've accepted the fact that this is it, I can pay my bills, and I've got a shilling or two in my purse . . . And that's all that matters to me . . . I'm easily pleased, I'm contented, and I think that goes a long way, doesn't it, being contented, if you're always wanting, you're never satisfied, your mind's working all the time . . . Got to have and . . . I'm not like that. I know I can't have it anyway, so what's the good in wanting? I don't want to be the richest woman in the churchyard, thank you very much . . . I want to be a happy and contented one now.

(Mrs F, in-depth)

Case 6.1 Mr M

Mr M is an example of how acceptance of situations and optimism helps one cope with major life events such as bereavement. He rated his QoL as very good, he was fit, and felt supported by his daughters and neighbours, although he was upset by the death of his wife a few years earlier. His daughters were important to him.

> Here, I have four daughters . . . They're all good, they ring me a couple of times a week. They're good daughters, I enjoy the company. They say to me, 'Can you manage Dad?' And I say, 'Of course I can.' That's my quality of life. It's a good one. If everyone else was as well, they wouldn't have any complaints.

However, one of the key factors bolstering him was his optimistic, opportunistic and easy-going personality, which he felt enabled him to focus on the positive parts of his life. For example, he missed his wife a great deal, but spoke of being content, if not happy:

> I: What makes you the most happy at the moment?
> R: I couldn't put it down to any single thing. I think I'm reasonably happy. I don't think I could ever be [really] happy again. I'm contented, that's a better word. I think I ceased being happy when I lost B [his wife] but I'm contented and that's enough.

He also missed being able to do things with his wife, such as going on holiday. However, instead he compensated and went on enjoyable group holidays, which also enabled him to meet new people:

> I've been [on coach holidays] twice by myself and the others were with friends. They're good value, extremely good value. The people are roughly about my age but they're not compelled to be. You get a five-day holiday, it's cheap, about £150, and it's a wonderful holiday. I've met lots of different people and I still meet them in town. I always stop and chat to them . . . The last time [I was on holiday] I went down to evening meal and there were three ladies who invited me over to sit with them. It was quite good. There was a lot of laughter and that's all that matters.

Mr. M suffered from arthritis, but he had taken steps to enhance his QoL with reflexology:

> I have a reflexologist, who comes to see me. She came yesterday, I could have floated when she did my feet and legs. She manipulates the toes and knees, I could have played football. [*laughter*] It's marvellous . . . she comes now every month . . . And on one day of that month I'm on top of the world [*laughs*].

> He said he had an adequate pension for his needs, but also made it clear that a good QoL is not about having a lot of money, but being able to afford what one would like to do, although he no longer had his wife to share enjoyment with, and missing her recurred throughout the interview:
>
> > Quality of life is enjoyment . . . I'm not well-off but I'm comfortable. So I don't have any money worries . . . The awful part about this is that I have money I can't spend because there's no enjoyment in spending it when you are on your own . . . I don't care how much money anyone has, I have sufficient, not wealthy by any means but I'm comfortable. I miss B just as much as when I lost her five years ago, you just learn to live with it . . . you can't do anything else . . . we were extremely close, we had a good marriage but now it is the thing that keeps me pretty well sane because in the evenings, especially the winter evenings, you are on your own . . .

Respondents frequently admitted to making downward social comparisons, comparing oneself with others worse off, to make themselves feel better about their own situations. These respondents tended to believe that people made their own QoL. For example:

When you look around, you think 'I've got troubles', then you look around and you see somebody else . . . in a wheelchair, and you think, 'Well, he's got troubles' . . . Quality of life is what you make it: you can't buy it, or inherit it, or anything like that, you know. So . . . as I say, it's what you make it . . . [QoL] is what you do yourself . . . Mine is to get out and about and do things for myself, or see things that I would like to see or haven't seen, you know . . . I don't expect to sit back and expect quality of life to come through the door.

(Mr V, in-depth)

Things that took quality away from life

Less than a fifth (17%) reported poor emotional well-being as taking quality from life, although 63% of in-depth respondents mentioned this. Respondents who scored as having psychological morbidity with the GHQ were more likely to mention poor psychological well-being taking quality away from life than those who did not report this: 25% and 14% respectively. There were no associations with having an optimistic or pessimistic disposition and mentioning this. Females were also more likely than males to report this theme: 20% and 13% respectively, although there was no difference by age or social class of respondent.

The reasons for reporting poor emotional well-being in relation to 'bad' QoL were said to be due mainly to declining health and loneliness, but also inability to do things after widow(er)hood, when taking on new (the deceased spouse's) tasks:

> I get frustrated when I can't do things – when the Hoover goes off – practical things that is. I find the gardening frustrating – been ripped-off so many times by so-called gardeners, this annoys me. It's the things my husband always did and took care of. Well, he's no longer here to do those kinds of things.

Poor emotional well-being was also mentioned in the context of fears for the future, including fears of losing health and independence. People greatly disliked the idea of being dependent on other people. The following two respondents voiced clearly the fear, which was expressed by several people, of giving up their home and entering care homes:

> I mean I often think well, what is there to look forward to in old age . . . it can be frightening if you think about it, you think of all these people and friends, of course, that have been ill, or are ill, or have died and you think oh, is this what's going to happen to us . . . the thing which would frighten me the most would be going in a home . . . I don't ever want to have to do that, having had . . . relatives – my mother went in a home . . . and then [*inaudible*]'s uncle and aunt who lived next door to each other, they had to go in . . . And we visited them for eleven years twice a week. Err, grandma died at a 101, and auntie died at 90 . . . It's a long life, and, err, we realised then what it would be like. Although they were very well looked after . . . I don't think their quality of life was very good . . . mentally they were both extremely alert . . . but . . . their bodies were just dying. And it's awful to watch it and to see it happening, especially when they're very alert, you know, and their bodies just give in.
>
> (Mrs A6, in-depth)

> *I*: And how would you describe the quality of your life at the moment?
> *R*: Well, I think I fear becoming infirm and having to depend on other people . . . or giving up, my home or anything like that; that really frightens me. I'd rather . . . die.
>
> (Mrs A4, in-depth)

Conclusion

Psychological outlook, including well-being was the sixth most frequently mentioned thing that gave life quality – 38% of survey respondents said this. And it was also one of the most frequently mentioned areas of QoL in the in-depth interviews. This suggests that QoL is strongly influenced by psychological outlook. Underlying respondents' mentioning of poor psychological well-being as taking quality away from life were adverse experiences, including illness or bereavement, and fears for the future. But respondents who mentioned psychological well-being as giving life quality often stressed the importance of employing coping strategies, including remaining positive and content, of acceptance and making the best of things. Psychological outlook (e.g. self-efficacy) also appeared to influence people's perceptions and coping strategies in the face of ill-health (for examples of these see Chapter 5), and may have health benefits.

However, there was evidence of social inequity, with those in higher socio-economic status groups having better psychological health and higher self-efficacy than those in lower groups. This supports other research which indicates that psychological outlook is associated with one's place in the status hierarchy (Marmot 2004). As was indicated in Chapter 1, the lower down the social scale one is, usually in relation to income group (wealth comparisons) or health status (health comparisons) then the opportunities for positive affect decrease and those for negative affect increase. It has been argued that for those in disadvantaged social positions, retirement and old age adds to their sense of powerlessness and loss of control (Phillipson 1987; Fennell *et al.* 1988). And as psychological resources were apparently important to QoL, there are inequities in the distribution of good QoL. This is an issue that has been neglected by positive psychologists.

Annex I: summary of sub-themes: psychological well-being

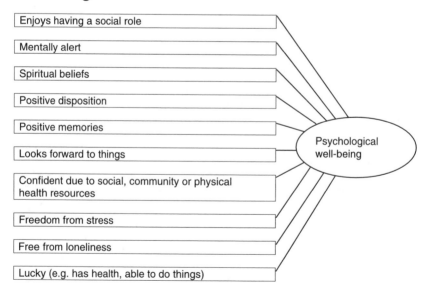

7

Social capital: home and neighbourhood

I think it's great because it is a little village and when you walk into the village everybody says 'Hello' and it's just great that people are so friendly, it's a super village, we've got a great little restaurant where you can meet friends and then come back and have coffee here, umm, it's idyllic really. In the past, I always seemed to live on the wrong side of the road or whatever, but now, thank God, it just seems to have fallen right for me.

I think one thing also for older people is that we would like more freedom from fear [*laughs*] round here especially. It looks very peaceful now, but we do have a lot of vandalism . . . and graffiti, and just recently I've had to replace my back rear fence because they came round in a car and . . . knocked it down . . .

So . . . you don't go nowhere. And I sit here at the top of this hill, in this flat, belonging to X council . . . I live here, there's just one [bus route], and if it doesn't want to run, it doesn't . . . And there's not just me on this road, there's more elderly . . . So you've got to walk up the hill because there's nothing to bring you, because the bus isn't there. And if it's winter, and it's icy, well you stay in, darling . . .

Given that the characteristics of the neighbourhood can constrain friendships and involvement in social activities, neighbourhood is theoretically associated with well-being of older people (Berkman and Glass 2000). The notions of social cohesion and wider social capital are only just beginning to be measured by social scientists in relation to health and older age. However, there is increasing interest among health researchers and social epidemiologists in broadening social measures to include social capital and social cohesion in order to study their effects on health status and mortality. Thus social capital is relevant to QoL also in relation to its enabling characteristics and its impact on health.

Neighbourhood disadvantage has been shown to be related to higher rates of death from cardiovascular disease (Roux *et al.* 2004), and analyses of routine indicators of urban environments (including health care, environmental quality, housing, urban clutter, local economy, income and education) have shown that these explained just over half of the variances in a health index (Takano and Nakamura 2001). Many such studies are likely to be reflecting the deleterious effects of material disadvantage on health. However, a critical review of 25 studies of the effect of local area social characteristics on individual health outcomes, adjusted for individual socioeconomic status, concluded that there was consistent evidence of modest neighbourhood effects on health (Pickett and Pearl 2001).

Neighbourhood-level socioeconomic status might influence health and mortality directly or indirectly through mechanisms such as available and accessible health services, information and education, healthy foods, environmental pollution, normative attitudes (e.g. towards health, smoking), social capital and support (Berkman and Glass 2000; Pickett and Pearl 2001). Ross and Mirowsky (2001) reported, on the basis of their multi-level modelling of results from a large population survey in Illinois, that residents of disadvantaged neighbourhoods had worse self-reported health and functional status, and more chronic health conditions than residents of more advantaged neighbourhoods. They found that the association was mediated by perceived neighbourhood disorder and fear (i.e. daily stress), and not health behaviours (e.g. level of outdoor physical activity). Their findings support the results of the other multi-level models they reviewed which indicated that neighbourhood disadvantage (or repeated exposure to threatening conditions) has a negative impact on health, by virtue of predisposing neighbourhoods to harmful conditions (e.g. disorder leading to fear and stress, with stress reducing immune response and release of stress hormones). Results suggest the impact is independent of the personal circumstances that lead individuals to live in disadvantaged areas.

It was pointed out in Chapter 1 that a cohesive community is marked by its connections between people (Kawachi and Berkman 2000), and its supportiveness; it is well endowed with stocks of social capital (Kawachi and Berkman 2000); it incorporates shared values, a sense of belonging to the community, trust and reciprocity. Social capital is a subset of social cohesion, and refers to the extent to which communities offer members opportunities, through involvement in social, recreational, voluntary and civic activities, and group membership, to increase their personal resources (Coleman 1988; Putnam 1995; Brissette et al. 2000). These can also all affect one's perceived autonomy and self-actualization and can act to improve the broader health of a community (Putnam 2000). The term social capital has also been used to refer to the collective value of all formal and informal social networks. However, the special significance of historical and present attachment to place of residence and neighbourhood among older people has been relatively neglected in its conceptualizations (Rubinstein and Parmelee 1992; Kellaher et al. 2004).

Commonly used indicators of social capital include community membership, trust, bonding, information flows, reciprocity and cooperation between people (Putnam 1995, 2000; Coulthard et al. 2001). High levels of broader social capital, like indicators of neighbourhood advantage (see p. 158), have been reported to be associated with lower mortality rates, better self-rated health, functional status and QoL (Kawachi et al. 1997a, 1997b, 1999; Grundy and Bowling 1999; Kawachi and Berkman 2000; Ross and Mirowsky 2001; Bowling et al. 2002a, 2003; Hyppa and Maki 2003), and with better psychological health (Lindeström 2004). Lower population density and ratings of better neighbourhood quality have also been reported to be associated with better health and QoL ratings (Cramer et al. 2004), and also with better self-rated health status (Kawachi et al. 1997a, 1997b, 1999; Kawachi and Berkman 2000). But relatively few investigators have fully explored the independent associations between social capital and physical health, mortality, psychological well-being or QoL (Brissette et al. 2000).

The survey

The questions on social capital in the survey questionnaire included a number of items from the British General Household Survey (Cooper et al. 1999; Coulthard et al. 2001; Walker et al. 2001). Areas with higher social capital were defined as those with more 'Very good' ratings for the quality of the area (facilities such as transport, shops, somewhere nice to go for a walk), fewer reported area problems (such as graffiti, noise, pollution), more ratings of 'Very safe' from crime and vandalism, and which were said to be neighbourly.

Social capital

The vast majority, 92%, of respondents said that they enjoyed living in their area of residence, although just 29% said they felt they could influence decisions in their area. Most, 74%, said they trusted most or many of the people in their neighbourhood, although 26% did not, or did not know people. Enjoyment of living in the area, and trust of other people in the neighbourhood, has been reported to increase with age in national surveys of all adults, reflecting longer length of residence with older age (Coulthard *et al.* 2001). However, while older people have high levels of area enjoyment and neighbourhood trust, these findings also indicate that a sizeable proportion of people are not integrated within their neighbourhoods – about four in ten people (43%) knew few or none of their neighbours, although just over half, 57%, said they knew most or many of the people. Coupled with the 26% (above) who did not trust or know people in their neighbourhood, these figures are of concern.

Just over half of respondents, 53%, rated their neighbourhoods as 'Very safe' and 35% as 'Fairly safe' to walk alone in during the daytime; 6% said it was 'A bit' to 'Very' unsafe and 6% never went out during the daytime. Just 12% rated their neighbourhoods as 'Very safe' to walk alone in after dark, 25% said it was 'Fairly safe', 21% felt it was 'A bit' to 'Very' unsafe and 42% never went out after dark.

Although a sizeable number considered their neighbourhoods to be generally unsafe at night, the vast majority of respondents did not have unreal expectations of their individual risks of assault or burglary being any higher than those of other men/women their age (it was shown in Chapter 6 that most people rated their chances of being mugged or burgled as the same, or even lower, than other people their age).

Very elderly people and women were the most likely to feel vulnerable. While there were no differences by age and feelings of being safe walking alone by day, people aged 75+ were more likely than those aged under 75 to report that they never went out during the day, reflecting their greater frailty and likely perception of vulnerability (11%:4% respectively). But the very elderly respondents were the least likely to feel safe walking alone at night. Just 26% of respondents aged 75+ said they felt safe walking alone at night, in comparison with 44% of those aged under 75 and 56% of people aged 75+ said they never went out after dark, in comparison with 34% of younger respondents.

In reflection of their poorer physical functioning (see Chapter 5), females were more likely than males to say they never went out during the day (11%:2% respectively), or after dark. Females were also less likely than males to report that they felt 'Very' or 'Fairly' safe walking alone at night (although not by day): 21%:55% respectively. This is comparable with other national statistics (Coulthard *et al.* 2001).

Respondents' neighbourhood safety ratings were not associated with the population density of the area, but were associated with Acorn affluence of area categories. For example, taking the combined area rating score (feeling safe day or night), just 12% of those who lived in thriving areas (wealthy suburbs) had 'very unsafe' area scores, compared with more of those in the striving areas (18%).

Most people rated the quality of the facilities in their area as either 'Very good', 'Good' or 'Average'. These included facilities for social and leisure activities, facilities for people aged 65+, rubbish collection, health services, transport, shops, and somewhere nice to go for a walk. The facilities which were most likely to be rated as 'Poor' or 'Very poor' were social and leisure facilities, facilities for people aged 65+, transport and closeness to shops (see Table 7.1). These are pertinent issues for older people, and areas of obvious relevance to local planning in relation to enhancing the social capital and cohesion of an area. The low ratings for social and leisure facilities and for facilities for people aged 65+ is a cause for concern given the expectation that community involvement leads to enhanced perceived autonomy and self-actualization. Less than half of respondents rated local transport as good at all. This, again, has implications for maintaining independence, social networks and participation in older age. Of course, these figures can only give a partial snapshot of the potential for community participation. For example, it was reported in Chapter 4 that there was a high level of social activity, and just under a fifth of respondents were engaged in voluntary work.

These items relating to the quality of the area were summed to produce an overall score: 13% of respondents scored their areas as 'Very good', 48% as 'Good', 39% fell into the middle, but 13% had 'Very poor' area ratings.

Table 7.1 Quality of area ratings (row %)

Quality of area rating (n = 994–5)	Very good/good	Average	Poor very poor	Don't know
Social and leisure activities	31	25	21	13
Facilities for people 65+	37	28	21	14
Rubbish collection	88	8	4	–
Local health service	82	12	4	2
Local transport	47	18	20	15
Closeness to shops	63	18	18	1
Somewhere nice to walk	72	14	12	2

Table 7.2 Problems within the area ratings (row %)

Problem rating (n = 994)	Very/fairly big problem	Minor problem	Happens but not a problem	Doesn't happen/apply to me	Don't know
Speed/volume of traffic	56	25	13	6	–
Noise	13	33	25	29	–
Crime	24	36	28	9	3
Air quality	11	28	19	37	4
Rubbish/litter	30	33	18	18	1
Graffiti	11	28	19	41	1

There was no association between social participation and ratings of the quality of public transport. However, engagement in social activities was associated with car access (and see Banister and Bowling 2004). There was a consistent trend with car access and number of social activities engaged in over the past month. For example, 49% of those who engaged in between 0 and 2 social activities had access to a car, compared with 67% of those who were engaged in between 3 and 4 and 82% of those who engaged in 5–12.

Table 7.2 shows that speed or volume of traffic, the amount of rubbish or litter and the amount of crime in an area were most likely to be rated as 'Very big' or 'Fairly big' problems (for between about a quarter and just over a half of respondents). These are all barriers to enablement. Rubbish and litter can be symptomatic of neglected areas, and may make people feel unsafe. Perceived high crime levels and fast traffic can combine with this to inhibit people from venturing out of their homes, especially at night.

These problem ratings were summed to form an overall score, which showed that 16% scored their areas overall as having very big problems, 21% fell into the middle, 59% scored minor problems and 4% scored no problems. People who lived in 'striving' Acorn areas were more likely than those who lived in more affluent areas to have the worst area problem scores: 24% in the worst two problem bandings scored <23 in comparison with 10% of those in the most affluent 'thriving' areas. This indicates that older people who live in poorer areas are the most likely to suffer from barriers to enablement and social engagement. This argument is illustrated by respondents themselves later in the chapter.

It appears that access to a car in the household is an important element of QoL in older age. In general, apart from the 6% who were housebound, most people aged 65 and over were active during the day, but after dark the situation was reversed, with little activity outside the home occurring in the evenings. People often expressed a high level of concern over traffic speed in their neighbourhoods. This, together with varying access to reliable public transport and, in particular, access to a car in the household, and fear of crime after dark, might explain their reduced activity. Neighbourhood safety, trust and engagement and access to transport were all important building blocks for a good, and independent, QoL in older age (Banister and Bowling 2004).

Associations with QoL

Association with QoL ratings

It would be expected that people who lived in more affluent areas, with good facilities, fewer social problems, where it was regarded as neighbourly and safe, would perceive their QoL to be higher, and this is illustrated in Table 7.3. This shows that those who rated the quality of the facilities in their neighbourhood as higher were more likely than those who gave them lower ratings to rate their QoL positively. The individual items relating to having good leisure facilities, rubbish collection, health services, transport, close-by shops and somewhere nice to go for a walk were all associated with positive QoL. Those who scored the neighbourliness of their areas as high were also more likely to have positive QoL ratings, and there was also a slight association with positive QoL and feeling safe. The table shows that, although those with the worst scores for area problems were less likely to rate their QoL positively, the trends between these variables were not always consistent, and this did not achieve statistical significance.

Trends with affluence of area were not all in a consistent direction, although those living in expanding areas (those populated with 'affluent executives/families, well-off workers/families') rather than aspiring areas ('new home owners, mature communities, white collar workers, better-off multi-ethnic areas') were more likely to rate their QoL higher. It is of interest that those who lived in the South East of England were most likely to rate their QoL positively, and those in London and in the South West were least likely to do so. The reasons underlying these differences are likely to be varied and include indicators of regional affluence, population density and so on.

The significant contribution of social capital to overall QoL is supported by the results of the regression modelling. It was reported in Chapter 3 that social

Table 7.3 Respondents' social capital characteristics by QoL rating (row %)

Social capital characteristics	So good it could not be better/very good/ good	Alright/bad/very bad/ so bad it could not be worse
Quality of facilities in area score (n = 994)		
<13 ('Very good')	90	10***
13–17	87	13
18–24	77	23
25–42 ('Very poor')	74	26
Area problem score+ (n = 993)		
<19 ('Very big problems')	72	28 ±
19–23	85	15
24–27	80	20
28–29	82	18
30 ('No problems')	86	14
Safety rating score (n = 993)		
<4 ('Very safe')	84	16*
3–4	85	15
5–8 ('Very unsafe')	77	23
0 ('Never go out')	62	38
Neighbourliness of area rating (n = 966)		
0 low	80	20*
1 high	85	15
Acorn category (affluence of area) (n = 970)		
Thriving	85	15**
Expanding	93	7
Rising	80	20
Settling	82	18
Aspiring	73	27

Striving	82	18
Grouped regions (n = 999)		
The North	81	19*
Midlands and East Anglia	81	19
London	77	23
South East	92	8
South West	78	22
Wales	81	19
Scotland	82	18

* p<0.05, ** p<0.01, *** p<0.001, ± not statistically significant (chi-square test); + Don't know/does not apply recoded to 0.

capital accounted independently for 2.1% of the variance in self-rated QoL. This may be a small proportion of the overall variance, but sizeable for quantitative indicators of subjective, amorphous concepts (QoL). The responses of older people reported in this chapter also emphasized the importance of the enjoyment of one's home and of living in a neighbourhood with good facilities, including transport, which is neighbourly, and where one feels safe.

Lay models

Things that gave life quality

Home and neighbourhood was mentioned as giving life quality by 37% of respondents. It was also mentioned by almost all (96%) of the in-depth interview respondents as giving life quality (see Chapter 3) (and see Annex I for summaries of the sub-themes). Living in a good neighbourhood (feeling safe, secure, friendly area, community feeling), having a good/friendly/helpful relationship with neighbours, and good local facilities (shops, markets, post office), including good services (street lighting, refuse collection, police, library, repairs), and having a pleasant landscape/surroundings were all said to be important to many respondents.

Respondents who mentioned their home and neighbourhood as giving life quality were more likely to be female than male: 41%:33% respectively, and to be aged 75 and over than under 75: 41%:34% respectively, possibly reflecting the greater amount of time women have traditionally spent at home compared to men, and the greater amount of time people in older age groups, and who are frailer, spend at home.

Mention of this theme as contributing to good QoL was associated with the population density of the area (numbers of people per hectare): 50% of those who lived in the least dense neighbourhoods (e.g. remote, rural areas) mentioned home and neighbourhood as part of a good QoL, in comparison with 29% of those in the most dense areas (e.g. built-up, inner-city housing) (the trends were consistent and in the expected direction for those in the other five population density groups).

In particular, and in support of the quantitative findings on area facilities and problem ratings (see p. 163), feeling safe and access to transport were said to be important for enabling people to retain their independence. These respondents clearly valued feeling safe, and also access to transport for enhancing their independence and QoL:

> Ah! Yes, living in a community where you feel safe. Yes nowadays all the news seems to be about old people being mugged or robbed and round here thankfully there is very little trouble like that.

> I think that we are lucky to get free prescriptions and free bus passes, and that doesn't worry you regarding expenses. With the bus pass you can get on and off as you like without paying and [it] saves my legs from walking. I'm happy that I can get about independently, and visit friends and that.

And, consistent with Chapter 4, neighbourliness was emphasized as important to QoL in older age, especially when people were frail or ill. In the place of having family living near by, neighbours could take on the role of providing security. This involved the reassurance that there was always someone looking out for them and someone who would help if it was needed. For example:

> Now my neighbours are marvellous . . . they're the ones who've put me into hospital three times and . . . well I wouldn't have been here if they hadn't been because I just wanted to sit here and go. But . . . they called the doctor and rushed me to hospital . . . My neighbours are very good. Them over there could be called at any time in emergency at any time. He watch me through my toilet window. If my toilet window is open, I'm out . . . my neighbour takes me to Sainsbury's every Tuesday, but Wednesday this week. But . . . he always takes me for the last three years, so I think that's very good of him.
>
> (Mrs E, in-depth)

Mr F was 76, and living with his wife who had problems with her eyesight. He worried about her health, but had neighbours he could call on for help:

So we've really got somebody we can knock, you know, if we're in trouble, we've got help . . . it's the quality of the neighbours I suppose, you've got to live with . . . they're ever so nice round this way . . . they're ready to help . . . it's the quality of life, as you say – the life, and that, and the people that actually live in your street.

Mr D valued the neighbourliness of his area. He could not get out a lot due to poor health and relied heavily on his neighbours for practical help, but reciprocal relationships were valued most:

I don't get out a great deal at all, I get out up to the post office on a Monday to draw my allowance, and my neighbour takes me to the supermarket every Friday to do a weekly shop . . . I'm fortunate in that I've got some good neighbours . . . who get me the odd things I want . . . Number ten takes me out shopping . . . and I wanted some cleaning of the gate, the hedge wanted doing and I got badly out of breath, so I asked him . . . 'Oh yes' he said, he'd [do] it. But . . . it's two way because I have a knowledge of electronics, and he'll come here with his little problems . . . and we get on well that way.

Other respondents emphasized their enjoyment of pleasant views, and areas in which to take 'nice walks', as well as the sense of belonging to a community and the enabling features of its facilities:

I: What do you think of when you hear the words 'quality of life'?
R: I think of here [C] actually. I think it's beautiful. It took me a long time, about 18 months to two years to accept the fact that I had retired. Once that happened I threw myself into the garden and bee-keeping. I do enjoy country life and ever since I moved down here, it's where I want to be . . .

(Mrs A2, in-depth)

I think it's great because it is a little village and when you walk into the village everybody says 'Hello' and it's just great that people are so friendly, it's a super village, we've got a great little restaurant where you can meet friends . . .

(Mrs A3, in-depth)

Wenger (1984b) found that elderly people who lived in rural areas where more likely than those who lived in urban areas to be more socially integrated in the community.

Things that took quality away from life

Almost a third of respondents, 30%, mentioned aspects of their home and neighbourhood as taking quality away from their lives, and 84% of in-depth respondents also mentioned this. This was associated with the perceived quality of the area (e.g. ratings of local facilities for people aged 65 and over, rubbish collection, health services, transport, shops and somewhere nice to go for a walk): 44% of survey respondents who rated their areas as very poor in relation to these facilities overall mentioned this theme, in comparison with 27% with middle ratings and 27% with very good ratings.

There was also an association with mention of this theme and overall problem ratings of the area (e.g. traffic, noise, rubbish, crime, graffiti and so on): 33% with 'Very big' problem scores for their area mentioned poor home and neighbourhood as taking quality away from life, in comparison with 30% of those with middle scores and 17% of those with 'No problem' scores. Respondents who felt unsafe walking alone in their neighbourhoods during the day (but not night) were more likely than those who felt safe, and those who never went out at night, to mention home and neighbourhood as taking quality away from life: 44%:29%:25% respectively. Poor neighbourhoods were seen as inhibiting social integration and participation, and creating feelings of insecurity. These respondents did not feel that their area was safe or friendly, or said that it lacked a community spirit. Some of them reported perceived danger from local vandals, groups of youths or gangs, damage to property, burglars and personal attack. Respondents also felt concern over the lack of a local police presence. Fear of crime and personal assault restricted these respondents' social activities, and many said they would not travel at night (see Case 7.1):

> Fear of crime is the first thing . . . we would like to go out in the evening but are frightened to do it . . . We would like to but would not travel on the metro at night.

> You've got to be careful when you go out at night, when I go out at night we drive around the block a couple of times before we actually go anywhere because everybody in the road's been burgled, everybody we know's had some sort of break-in in the last few years . . . so it's all that sort of thing . . . I mean you look at people walking by, young people – could be perfectly innocent, but you're thinking I wonder if he's been in my house? You know, when you've been burgled three times like we have here . . . so – it made us frightened of going out for, for a while, you know . . . I'm sitting at the pub having a pint and I'm thinking there's somebody breaking, kicking my door in [*laughs*] so . . . that period was a bad time . . . Wife crying and all that sort of business, you know . . . so it's all that sort of thing . . . that we worry about at our age.
>
> (Mr U, in-depth)

> I wouldn't want to go out in the evenings anyway . . . Not round here. We've had an old lady up the street over there . . . at twenty to nine in the morning was mugged,

she was pushed face down, her face was in a terrible, terrible state – for eight pounds, and she had her hip broken, but she's 86 – she was off to B [Europe] in two days, but she couldn't get there . . . I don't feel safe, that is one drawback [to my QoL], I just don't feel safe . . . it's the same old story, you never see the police . . . and they said they would make their presence felt after that happened to J, but, but I've never seen one . . . but it does help an older person if they can see there is someone there who can help them . . . our generation are used to seeing the police about . . . And I think it helps a lot, gives you that little bit of confidence . . . I carry an alarm . . . I don't know if it'd do any good, but it gives me a bit of confidence.

(Mrs F, in-depth)

Case 7.1 Mrs J

Mrs J was aged 73 and had been widowed twice. She rated her QoL as 'Very good' at her baseline QoL interview. She was in good physical health and enjoyed going swimming and keeping fit. However, despite this, and after being burgled when she was in the house, she said she suffered from depression and was now taking anti-depressants, which she was anxious to stop taking. Fear of crime still affected Mrs J's life, as did youth vandalism, because her garage was often painted with graffiti.

> I think one thing also for older people is that we would like more freedom from fear [*laughs*] round here especially. It looks very peaceful now, but we do have a lot of vandalism . . . and graffiti, and just recently I've had to replace my back rear fence because they came round in a car and . . . knocked it down . . . if we perhaps had more presence of the police round the area, but . . . that would sort of be a bit of a deterrent anyhow – I can't say they'd stop it, but . . . it would certainly make everyone think that someone was sort of watching . . . [*laughs*] . . . I mean . . . where I lived with my second husband, we were burgled three times. Yeah, the last one was the worst because my husband had died and I was living alone in the bungalow . . . they kicked the front door in . . . I was asleep in bed, and I woke up to all this happening. I've been on the anti-depressants since then, because I can't really get over it. It's not very pleasant . . .

But QoL is multi-faceted. Life events and losses in older age can be cumulative, and her depression was also contributed to by bereavement, and the loss of her friends, which contributed to her worry about what might happen to her:

> She was my neighbour where I lived before. She fell and broke her hip, and she was in hospital and she died on . . . so she was in hospital quite a long time. I used to go

and visit her, and I found that terribly depressing because she was in a ward with a lot of very elderly people, and she was so unhappy there. That was half the trouble there. She had about three [infections] whilst she was in there, she had pneumonia which she died from in the end. She had an infection in her hip and all sorts of things . . . she got over the actual operation very well, and they wouldn't send her out because she had no one to look after her and so they kept her in, but in doing so she caught all these other infections and she died in the end. That really upset me. The other friend I'd known for years too . . . he had been in hospital . . . for nine weeks with some heart problem, and they really did nothing apart from change his tablets all the time. And eventually they discharged him, and about three weeks after . . . I invited them for a meal and he wasn't too bad . . . and then the next day his wife phoned to say that he'd died in the night. I was awfully worried, but he'd had another heart attack. So that was a terrific shock to the system really . . .

(See p. 132 for fuller case)

Other problems mentioned included difficulties with neighbours (e.g. noisy neighbours, anti-social behaviour by children), poor local facilities (e.g. shops) and poor local services (e.g. police, repairs, street lights, refuse collection, social work). Some people said they were 'stressed' by their homes due to repairs that were needed, and household chores that respondents found difficult. As Walker and Walker (2005) stated, housing is very important to older people's QoL, because they spend more time at home than younger people. But home maintenance and repairs can also pose increasing problems for people who are less physically able.

Fears for the future and losing independence were sometimes heightened when people lived in areas with poor social resources and public services. Lack of easy access to reliable, cheap and convenient public transport was mentioned as inhibiting social contacts and activities. Some of these respondents said that it was more difficult to get out and about because of inadequate transport, uncomfortable buses with high steps, or difficulties walking to bus stops. Some respondents spoke of expensive fares for short distances, which they could not afford. Not all local authorities offered free or discounted travel for retired people. And even where authorities reduced fares by about a third for older people, this can still be expensive for them:

So . . . you don't go nowhere. And I sit here at the top of this hill, in this flat, belonging to X council . . . I live here, there's just one [bus route], and if it doesn't want to run, it doesn't ... And there's not just me on this road, there's more elderly ... So you've got to walk up the hill because there's nothing to bring you, because the bus isn't there. And if it's winter, and it's icy, well you stay in, darling. That's when you rely on your children ... But the bus fares are atrocious. I mean it's nearly £1 to go up – so that's taking £2, if you go there and come back, that's £2 ... Not everybody's got £2 to spare, love ... so it's all wrong.

(Mrs M, in-depth)

Awareness of poor public transport facilities in their areas also led people to value their continued ability to drive their cars for their enjoyment and independence:

Public transport is not good so I worry about getting around as I get older, especially as our friends are scattered – whilst we can drive there is no problem.

The car – it makes my quality of life. It allows me to travel to our caravan, to get out to the seaside ... I am unable to walk far due to breathing problems and the car gives me independence to get about.

Other respondents mentioned poor local services and community facilities in general as adversely affecting QoL. Some added that they wanted more provision of social activities for older people, and educational and exercise classes, which were close enough for them to attend.

Conclusion

Almost all respondents said they enjoyed living in their area, and there was a high level of neighbourhood trust. The British General Household survey also found that older people were more likely than younger people to report that they enjoyed living in their area and to know more of their neighbours (in reflection of their length of residence). However, about four in ten people also said they knew few people, or no one in their neighbourhoods. And only just over half of respondents rated their areas as 'Very safe'. In addition, about a fifth of people who went outdoors felt unsafe, and about four in ten people said they never went out after dark. Large national surveys have also reported that older people and women were the groups most likely to say they felt 'Very unsafe' walking alone after dark (Coulthard et al. 2001). In addition, the government's Citizenship Surveys (Attwood et al. 2003) found that the majority of people of all ages in England and Wales feel unsafe walking alone in their neighbourhoods at night, again, especially older people and women. Feeling safe is important for people, and in particular for older people's QoL.

171

It has direct relevance at national and local government levels for policy and planning.

This study also found a consistent trend with car access and number of social activities engaged in over the past month. Transport is important in terms of facilitating access to local facilities, leisure activities and social participation. It is an important part of social capital in maintaining social relationships – essential building blocks of QoL (Chapter 3). Travel by car is likely to increase given the growth in car ownership by older people (see Banister and Bowling 2004). However, one of the greatest areas of concern in relation to neighbourhoods related to the speed and volume of traffic. This is an issue of obvious policy relevance.

Most people aged 65 and over were active during the day, but after dark the situation was reversed, with little activity outside the home occurring in the evenings. Concern about traffic speed, access to a car in the household, varying levels of access to good public transport and fear of crime after dark might explain reduced activity. Neighbourhood safety, trust and engagement, and access to transport were all important building blocks for a good, and independent, QoL in older age (Banister and Bowling 2004). The low ratings respondents gave to the social and leisure facilities in their areas, and for facilities for people aged 65+ is also a cause for concern. In addition, less than half of respondents rated local transport as good at all. The implication is that communities are inadequate in their provision of facilities for the promotion of social activity and leisure, and local transport is failing to help older people retain their independence and participation in society.

In sum, home and neighbourhood are important to people. They were mentioned as giving life quality by over a third of respondents, and by almost everyone at their in-depth interviews. In addition, social capital was an independent predictor of self-rated QoL. Living in a good neighbourly area, feeling safe, with good facilities, including transport, is important for QoL. However, there was obvious room for improvement at local levels, in particular of facilities to promote social activity, perceptions of safety and local transport.

Annex I: summary of sub-themes: home and neighbourhood

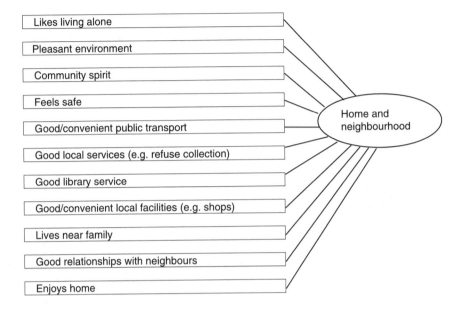

8

Financial circumstances and having enough money

Having my health and having a reasonable standard of living. Well they both give you the freedom to do what you want. You are not dependent on anyone.

The quality of life has deteriorated financially year by year from pensions. The annual increases are not nearly enough . . . The increases in fuel have caused financial problems. I have had to let my allotment go as I cannot afford to do anything. I am prevented travelling as much as I used to or would like.

In Britain, the largest source of income for people of state pension age is state benefits, including the state retirement pension. While the vast majority of men of pensionable age receive the full state pension, less than half of women receive this, probably because of reduced national insurance contributions while child-rearing. In 2002–3, the state pension comprised about half of the income for a single, non-cohabiting pensioner or a couple where the man (traditionally defined as 'head of household') has reached state pension age, occupational pensions made up just over a quarter, and tiny proportions were made up from earnings, investment income and other types of income (Office for National Statistics 2004).

In 1979, just under half of pensioners in Britain were in the bottom fifth of the net equivalized income distribution, but by 2002–3 this proportion had almost halved to about a quarter. Single female pensioners were the most likely to be in the bottom fifth, and single male pensioners in the top fifth; older pensioners were also most likely to be at the bottom end of the distribution (Office for National Statistics 2004). It has been estimated that poverty affects around a fifth of all people of pensionable age (New Philanthropy Capital 2004). For most, retirement and older age is a period of declining living standards, especially with the decline in the basic state pension since 1984 relative to average earnings (Walker 1993; Bond and Corner 2004). And older women, who are less likely than men to have an occupational pension, or to receive the full state pension, are even worse off.

Because of the extremes in financial circumstances in older age, reporting has tended to emphasize either the affluence or poverty of life after retirement. For example, Age Concern England (2004), in an attempt to promote a more positive view of older age, stated that people aged over 50 own 80% of the personal assets in the UK, hold 60% of the savings and account for 40% of consumer spending. And certainly, it is likely that the *next* generation of people living on retirement pensions will be better off in terms of financial reserves, even if their pensions fall short of expectations. Estimates suggest that people aged over 45 are responsible for almost 80% of the financial wealth and 30% of consumer spending (Harkin and Huber 2004). But in contrast, a national survey of 10,000 people aged over 60 carried out by Help the Aged (Wright 2004), funded by British Gas, reported that 58% dreaded the onset of winter because of fears about money, illness and isolation. One in three of those questioned expressed fears about winter heating bills. Just over half (51%) said they had to manage on less than £8000 a year, and only 12% said they had annual incomes in excess of £18,000. Neither perspective is incorrect, but they need balancing. It needs to be remembered that while a large number of people who have occupational pensions are better off in retirement than previous generations, this still leaves around a fifth to a quarter of people on pensions in Britain who live in relative poverty.

It was described in Chapter 1 that older people in advanced industrial societies hold the state responsible for their marginalization from social and economic life, especially through traditional, age-based, state retirement policies (see Grundy and Bowling 1997). While by no means a new phenomenon, the problem is that, for most individuals, the timing of their retirement is not within their control. The potential stress of retirement needs to be seen in the context of social position. People who reach retirement are the survivors, given that those in lower socioeconomic groups are well documented to be more likely to die earlier than those in higher socioeconomic groups (Townsend and Davidson 1982; Whitehead 1987). And the experience of retirement itself is partly dependent on accumulated savings, and adequacy of income from pensions, which are also class related (Taylor and Ford 1983). Even though research has long shown that people value the freedom of retirement (Crawford 1972), it has also shown that people in the lower social classes have few resources to spend on leisure activities in retirement, in contrast to those in the middle classes, who have the social and financial resources built up over a lifetime, which can be used to enhance their activities in retirement (Guillemard 1982). Fennell *et al.* (1988) and Phillipson (1987) argued that for those in disadvantaged social positions, retirement and old age adds to their sense of powerlessness and loss of control. There are also well-established associations between individual indicators of socioeconomic position and health (Robert and House 1996). Level of income over one's life, for example, affects the type of food consumed, clothing, housing and opportunities across life. These areas can all have an impact on health. More recent approaches have emphasized more positive images of ageing, citing concepts of disability-free life expectancy, and data on the increasing wealth of retired people who have occupational pensions. But Blane *et al.* (2004) have pointed out that such models, rather than conflicting, can be seen as ideal type opposites on a spectrum. This is supported by the data on retirement income.

Although current income inevitably affects lifestyle in retirement, there is less consensus about the influence of life course socioeconomic position or income on perceived QoL. Blane *et al.* (2004), reporting on longitudinal data from a sample of about 300 people, argued that perceived QoL (measured using a scale of self-efficacy) in early old age appeared to be influenced primarily by current contextual factors, such as material circumstances (housing tenure and receipt of means-tested welfare benefits) and serious health problems, rather than life-course influences (the latter were limited to shaping people's circumstances in later life). In contrast, Breeze *et al.* (2004), reporting data from a large cluster randomized controlled trial of the care of older people in primary care found that having a low socioeconomic position in middle age as well as in older age exacerbated the risk of poor QoL (measured using four dimensions of functioning from the Sickness Impact Profile and the Philadelphia Geriatric Morale Scale).

Objective indicators, such as income, are usually significantly but weakly correlated with overall happiness, well-being, life satisfaction and perceived QoL probably because QoL reflects the sum of objective indicators and subjective perceptions (Saris 1996; Bowling and Windsor 2001; Bowling and Gabriel 2004). People are apparently happier if they live in wealthy rather than poor nations (Diener and Biswas-Myers 2002), and levels of happiness, satisfaction and other indicators of QoL increase with level of income (Veenhoven 1991; Heylighen and Bernheim 2000). But once a certain basic level of human need has been met in a society (Maslow 1968), and a certain level of wealth has been achieved, material wealth seems to contribute relatively little to greater happiness (James 1997, 2003) and may even have the reverse effect (Kasser 2002). Although this relativist perspective is contentious, there is supportive evidence (see Chapters 1 and 6). It has been suggested that one of the main psychological strategies for maintaining well-being, and promoting self-mastery and control is the use of self-enhancing social comparisons (Ryff 1999). If people make upward comparisons of themselves and their circumstances with others who are better off, then they are more likely to be unhappy, dissatisfied with their lot and have unmet expectations than people who make downward comparisons with others who are worse off.

The survey

The circumstances and characteristics of respondents were measured using standard ONS Omnibus Survey measures, covering gross annual income, paid work, socioeconomic group (social class was coded using both the old and newer classifications), housing tenure, car ownership, age of leaving full-time education, highest educational qualifications and type of area of residence (population density per hectare, and Acorn classification of affluence). There is known to be a socioeconomic gradient in morbidity and mortality, regardless of which indicator of socioeconomic status is used (Yngwe et al. 2001). Level of education, as an indicator of success in life, would normally be expected to predict occupational class, income, housing tenure and type of housing. But it is particularly important to use multiple measures of current socioeconomic position in studies of older age, given the debate about the sensitivity of individual socioeconomic indicators in retired populations, the majority of whom experience a drop in income upon retirement, with few members of the current generation of retired people having enjoyed the benefits of higher education (Grundy and Holt 2001; Bowling 2004b).

The characteristics of respondents were described in Chapter 2, and these are summarized in Box 8.1.

Income drops for most people in older age. Dependency on pensions is reinforced as any financial assets they may have become depleted. It was pointed out in Chapter 2 that respondents' general lack of qualifications had repercussions, not just for their main occupations and income when working, but also for their retirement income. Almost half had an annual income of less than £6240, reflecting their reliance on state pensions. And almost a third of respondents still had sizeable outgoings in their retirement as they either rented their homes or were still paying off their mortgages.

Box 8.1 Socioeconomic characteristics of respondents

- Just under half (48%) had left school at or before the age of 14 (n = 486), or had no formal education (n = 5).
- Most, almost two-thirds (64%), had no formal qualifications.
- Almost half (47%) were in the lower socioeconomic classes (old social class coding).
- A small number (5%) were in paid work.
- Over two-thirds (67%) had access to a car or van in the household.
- Almost half (47%) reported having an annual income of less than £6240, just over a fifth (22%) reported having £6240<£9360 and almost a third (31%) reported having between £9360 and £17,680+.
- Just over three-quarters (76%) owned their own home outright or on a mortgage.
- Just over a third (35%) (n = 352) lived in the two lowest population density bands, while, at the other extreme, about a quarter (24%) lived in the two highest population density bands.
- Just over a quarter (26%) lived in areas classified as 'thriving', 15%, at the other extreme, lived in 'striving' areas.

A commonly used indicator of social deprivation is access to a car or van within the household. A third of respondents had no access to a car or van. However, as has been illustrated throughout this book, this was due to a mixture of reasons, and not just economic (e.g. people had to give up driving for health reasons, and widows were often without a car once their husbands had died as they had never learnt to drive). But, as illustrated in Chapters 6, 7 and 9, access to transport was often vital for retaining social participation and independence and maintaining a sense of self-efficacy. Many people commented that they either had no access to good public transport or they did not feel safe using public transport at night in their neighbourhoods, and were thus effectively isolated (see Chapter 7). This is perhaps unsurprising given the sizeable numbers who lived in either remote areas or dense, inner-city areas.

Despite their low levels of income, it was shown in Chapter 6 that between 42 and 53% of respondents felt they were better off than other people like themselves, or than they had expected, in general and than when they were younger ('in your 40s'). Just 15 to 28% said they felt worse off. Given the low level of income of almost half the sample, these expectations and comparisons are likely to reflect low financial expectations for older age, rather than reflecting having adequate finances.

Associations with QoL

Associations with QoL ratings

Table 8.1 shows that all socioeconomic indicators, except income, were associated with more positive QoL ratings. Of course, access to a car or van might also reflect the contribution this made to people's independence and ability to get out and about, and hence their QoL (see Chapters 6 and 9). Although those with the highest incomes were the most likely to rate their lives positively, the trends with income and QoL rating were not all consistent, and did not achieve statistical significance (see Bowling *et al.* 2002a). Income also failed to achieve statistical significance in the regression model of independent predictors of QoL ratings (see Chapter 3 and below).

In support of social comparisons theory, however, and as reported in Chapter 6, people were more likely to rate their QoL as good in some degree, if their financial and living circumstances were better than they had expected they would be, and if they were thought to be better than other people's (of the same age). Chapter 6 also showed that those with highest (best) overall expectations and comparisons scores were more likely to rate their overall QoL positively. This indicates the importance of social comparisons for one's well-being and self-esteem.

Despite their significance (except income) at the bivariate level of analysis, it was shown in Chapter 3 that adding the main socioeconomic indicators (social class, income, housing tenure, education) into the model of QoL explained just 1% of the variance in QoL ratings, and these socioeconomic variables all lost statistical significance in the model. On the other hand, as again shown in Chapters 3 and 6, social comparisons and expectations were significant in the model, and explained a greater proportion of self-evaluated QoL than objective indicators of socioeconomic status and income. This supports a relative deprivation model.

Lay models

Things that gave life quality

Having no financial worries about bills or debts, having enough money for essentials, being able to afford to run/maintain a car/pay for petrol was mentioned by 33% of respondents as giving quality to life ('Good'). It was also mentioned by almost three-quarters (73%) of the in-depth interview respondents as giving life quality (see Annex I for examples of the sub-themes).

Table 8.1 Respondents' socioeconomic characteristics by QoL rating (row %)

Socioeconomic characteristics	So good it could not be better/ very good/good	Alright/bad/very bad/so bad it could not be worse
Social class (old coding) (n = 999)		
I (professional)	90	10**
II (intermediate)	87	13
IIInm (skilled non manual)	82	18
IIIm (skilled manual)	75	25
IV (partly skilled)	76	24
V (unskilled)	87	13
Armed forces	−+	−
Never worked/inadequate	92	8
Social class (new coding) (n = 972)		
Employers and managers, large organizations	88	12**
Higher professionals	90	10
Lower managerial, professional	88	12
Intermediate occupations	85	15
Small employers, own account workers	75	25
Lower supervisory, crafts etc.	76	24
Semi-routine occupations	77	23
Routine occupations	79	21
Gross annual income (n = 952):		
<£4160	81	19±
£4160<£9360	79	21
£9360>£17,680	84	16
£17,680+	90	10
Housing tenure (n = 997)		
Owns outright	85	15*
Owns on mortgage	88	12
Rents local/housing association	72	28
Rents privately	72	28

Age left full-time education (n = 998)		
Up to 14	78	22*
15–18	85	15
19–25	90	10
25+	85	15
Highest education qualification (n = 999)		
Degree, higher degree	91	9*
Higher education below degree	91	9
A levels or higher	87	13
ONC/BTEC, O level/GCSE equivalent	90	10
GCSE grade D-G.CSE 2–5 or standard, other qualifications	85	15
No formal qualifications	78	22
Car or van available to household (n = 999)		
Yes	87	13***
No	72	28

+ 100% but total = 2, calculation of percentages not appropriate
*p<0.05, **p<0.01, ***p<0.001, ± not statistically significant (chi-square test)

Mention of financial situation as giving life quality was more likely to be made by men than women: 38%:27% respectively; and by respondents aged under 75 than 75 and over: 36%:27% respectively. Respondents in the higher social classes I to IIInm were also more likely to mention this than respondents in lower social classes IIIm to V: 35%:30% respectively, probably reflecting the higher incomes they enjoyed. The contrast was strongest comparing the professional social class I group (42% mentioned this theme) with the unskilled social class V group (26% mentioned this theme). Accordingly, respondents who received the highest incomes (mainly in the form of retirement pensions) were the most likely to mention finances as contributing to their good QoL: 54% of those with £17,680+ per annum said this, in comparison with 45% of those with £9360<£17,680, 26% of those with £4160<£9360 and 25% of those with less than £4160.

The responses of those in the lower income groups sometimes reflected low expectations and feelings that their income was adequate if they could 'get by' and 'pay off debts'. In contrast, those in the higher income groups sometimes emphasized enjoyment and the importance of sufficient funds for continued participation in society – to enable them to do what they wanted, especially for pastimes and going away (generally called 'luxuries'). A few respondents referred to their income as adequate or favourable relative to others who were perceived to be worse off, with their parents or themselves in the past when worse off, representing downward health and wealth comparisons (there were no upward comparisons). For example, one woman whose annual income was between £14,500 and £20,000, said: 'Having sufficient income to do what I want . . . Having enough money – without being rich – makes me privileged compared with my parents.'

Others said that they appreciated having sufficient money for basic living and leisure needs (e.g. to run the car, to pay bills, to have holidays) so they did not have to 'worry' about money and bills, for example, as this man, who lived on an income of between £6500 and £7500, said:

> [it's] having sufficient money, I mean not excessive money, just enough to do what you require, run your car, say, and pay your bills, and have the odd holiday. I don't mean thousands of pounds or millions of pounds, but sufficient money not to have to worry about money.
>
> (Mr I, in-depth)

And Mrs F, although having an annual income of between £4500 and £5500, was simply content to not be in debt and to be able to afford to pay her bills. She justified her low financial expectations by referring to her life course and the lack of money in the family when she was growing up, her outlook of acceptance of situations and general satisfaction with life, which was helped by having the security of her home:

> As a family we never had a lot, my dad died when we were little tots, so we've never [had] a lot of money in the family, so I've never been one that's [been] brought up to want, you know. I mean I've got neighbours and friends . . . they've got to have this, they've got to have that . . . For me, there's a lot of things I would like, but I can't afford them, so I've accepted the fact that this is it.

But having sufficient money was an instrument which enabled people to do the things they liked doing (i.e. empowered them), as Mrs I, who had an income of between £5500 and £6500, indicated:

> I: What would improve the quality of your life?
> R: Not much really. I have this house, I've got my health, I don't have loads of money but I've got enough to do what I want to do . . . Health is supreme. Health, friends and enough money. As I said before, those three things must be there to enjoy life. If you don't have that there is no purpose. With those, you are empowered to do as you so wish.

Respondents who had additional pensions to their state pension often stated that they felt 'lucky'. For example, Mrs J downwardly compared her own financial situation, which was bolstered by her spouse's occupational pension to take it up to between £9500 and £10,500, with those of her friends who were living on a state pension:

> I'm fairly fortunate, I've been able to live quite happily and go on holidays and things [*laughs*] which a lot of old people can't, especially those who only have their state pension – I don't know how they cope, to be honest . . . I know we've had the five pound rise . . . But then the council tax goes up, and TV licences go up, everything goes up – five pounds really goes nowhere [*laughs*] but as I say I'm fortunate, I have a work pension, and I have half of my husband's work pension, so, I, I'm not too bad, but, it, I do feel sorry for a lot of my friends, I know they really are hard up.
>
> (Mrs J, in-depth)

Things that took quality away from life

Not having enough money was mentioned as a 'bad' area of QoL by almost a quarter, 23%, of respondents and just over half, 53%, of the in-depth respondents mentioned this. Inadequate finances taking quality away from life was more likely to be mentioned by men than women, possibly reflecting traditional role divisions and the male responsibility for household finances: 26%:19% respectively. It was also more likely to be mentioned by younger respondents aged under 75 than those aged 75+: 26%:17% respectively. These findings reflect the author's earlier research on the important things in life to people (Bowling 1995a, 1995b). However, mention of this theme (as 'bad') was not significantly associated with social class or annual income, possibly because most respondents had a relatively low level of income, and possibly in part support of social comparisons theory (see Chapter 6). Perceptions of satisfaction and adequacy may partly depend on what people have relative to a norm, which is affected by what others have.

Although mention of finances as contributing to bad QoL was not associated with level of income, an inadequate standard of living was reported by the respondents who said that not having enough money took quality away from their lives. While it may be argued that major expenses, such as mortgage payments, are generally reduced or removed in older age, other expenses can increase if health and functioning worsens (e.g. the need for domestic help or special furniture or fittings; or extra heating, especially by those who no longer go out at night and/or during the day). Although social services departments in local authorities can provide social care, not everyone on low incomes qualifies for free help, or can afford the sliding scale of charges (depending on income, savings and investments). While some people were upset that they could not afford to buy new furniture, or that they could not afford to decorate their homes, several said they could not afford sufficient domestic help which they needed due to declining health and mobility.

For example, Mrs N, who was a 71-year-old widow, said she was lonely, and that her QoL was very poor. She spoke about both her poor health and financial problems as affecting her QoL. Due to dizziness, she had suffered from accidents while carrying out household tasks such as cooking. Her poor health prevented her from decorating her home and tending to her garden, yet she could not afford to pay someone else to do these things for her, and sometimes went short of food. Her annual income was between £7000 and £8500: 'I mean my money doesn't always stretch out, now. And there's some weekends . . . that I end up with perhaps a fiver in my pocket, and I've got to feed myself for a week on that, you know'.

The importance to frail older people of being able to afford suitable furniture is illustrated by Mrs Q who was living in sheltered housing, and dependent just on her state pension. She spoke of how new furniture would help her to retain her independence:

> *I:* And you . . . said you'd like your finance to be a bit better. What would you do?
> *R:* I should buy myself one of those adjustable beds. And a chair that I could stand up [from] easily. And ahh . . . I should have some cupboards, in my bedrooms . . . that would make life easier. Well, I'm talking millionaire, now: I would like a bath that you could get into easier, and all things that . . . I could be independent until . . . the rest of my days.

People on low incomes are unable to build up savings or other economic resources to bolster their retirement income. Among those with some savings, there were concerns about them being depleted over time. As this married woman, whose joint pension was still under £15,000, said: 'Our income is static – we might have to worry in the future, depending on how long we live.'

Others were worrying about not being able to afford major household maintenance bills (e.g. for a replacement gas central heating/water boiler, replacing tiles which had blown off the roof, leaking drainpipes and so on). They commented that they had few, or no, surplus funds available to pay for these (see Case 8.1).

Several people said that their state pension was inadequate to meet their basic needs; they were not only worried about paying bills, but they could not afford

---

Case 8.1 Mrs O

Mrs O was a widow. She said her QoL was good overall, but adversely affected at times by her caring role and not having enough money. She spent much of her time caring for other people, including an elderly aunt, and her grandchildren. She had also looked after her husband before he died. She viewed her responsibility for her aunt as somewhat of a burden, and at times she found herself providing a lot of the childcare for her grandchildren, one of whom was asthmatic. In addition, Mrs O's QoL was affected negatively by her financial situation, as she was living just on the state pension. She described the things she would like to be able to afford and how difficult it is to live on the state pension, especially with household repairs to do:

> . . . but they [the firemen] went all round the house to check up for me, to make sure that I'd got proper windows . . . you really ought to have a new window in here, the fireman said, because it's not safe, so I rang – now I'm getting that sorted out, that's another [thing] . . . Well, it was rotting, and he said it was too dangerous, so I ought to get that changed. So that's what I mean, one thing on top of the other . . . and the boiler went, heating up the water – then the fridge packed up . . . sometimes I wish I could win the lottery . . . that would sort it all out, the money problems . . . I just have to be extra careful . . . Like people say how can you live without central heating? . . . if you never have it you never miss it. Yeah . . . that would be nice . . . Nice not to worry . . . that would be lovely . . . I'd like to win the lottery, there's so much you could do with it . . . I just, be grateful for what I've got.

---

luxuries such as outings or holidays. Some respondents felt that they simply could not afford to enjoy life:

> *I:* And you mentioned not enough money – what kind of things would you buy . . .?
> *R:* Well, I'd have a holiday for a start . . . a good thing would be to be able to go to the cinema, I can't remember the last time I went there, or, well, or theatrical, or – or a train ride, or little things that needs money . . . Can't do anything on £53 a week . . . It's not enough . . . to really enjoy life. I mean it's enough to get through, but what can you do . . . But you know, we all pull together, me and [*inaudible*] me husband . . . we just get through . . . but nothing spare . . . So, I mean that does affect your life. If you've got money you can move, can't you – even if you're not very good on your legs you can order taxis like you did . . . You can't do that on what I get.

> (Mrs R, in-depth)

Some respondents commented that they could no longer afford to drive their cars, or travel by car or public transport so often, which adversely affected their QoL (see also Chapter 9):

> The quality of life has deteriorated financially year by year from pensions. The annual increases are not nearly enough . . . The increases in fuel have caused financial problems. I have had to let my allotment go as I cannot afford to do anything. I am prevented travelling as much as I used to or would like. I am missing out three journeys to my caravan in the six month season.

> . . . more pension would help me to be able to enjoy myself more. I have to keep using my nest egg to have the jobs around the house done, and I have no way of building me nest egg up. Finance is the top thing really.

Conclusion

Almost half of the respondents to this survey reported having an annual income of less than £6240. At the other end of the scale, almost a third (31%) (299) reported having an income of between £9360 and £17,680+. However, few, just over a fifth, said they were worse off than they had expected to be, which is likely to reflect people's low expectations for old age.

Although income did not retain statistical significance in the regression model of independent predictors of QoL, adequacy of finances was mentioned by a third of survey respondents, and almost three-quarters of in-depth interview respondents, as giving quality to life ('Good'). About a quarter of survey respondents, and about half of in-depth interviewees, mentioned not having enough money as taking quality away from their lives.

Mention of finances as giving life quality was associated with annual income, although there was no association between mention of finances as taking quality away from life and income. Money was said by these respondents to be important to QoL, not just in terms of ensuring basic needs were met, but in enabling people to participate in society, to enjoy themselves and to free them from worry about paying bills, having enough money to meet emergencies, or paying for practical help when needed.

It is possible that in older age, when incomes are more levelled due to people's reliance on pensions, objective indicators of financial status are less sensitive than subjectively perceived financial circumstances, which, in turn, may be influenced by social expectations and comparisons. It has been shown elsewhere that quantitative socioeconomic indicators are not necessarily sensitive measures of socioeconomic position in retirement (Grundy and Holt 2001; Bowling 2004b). The importance of perceptions, rather than sole reliance on objective indicators, is given further support by the finding that financial social comparisons and expectations were among the main explanatory variables of QoL self-ratings in the regression model (see Chapters 3 and 6). Satisfaction and happiness, it appears, can partly depend on what people have relative to a norm, affected by what others have (see Chapters 1 and 6).

However, it should be cautioned that policy-making should not be based simply on satisfaction with one's lot, especially in older age groups, where perceptions are likely to be based on low expectations. One's psychological outlook is also shaped by social position (Marmot 2004 and see Chapter 6). This study does have implications for the design of measurement instruments: perceptions are important to tap, but alongside objective indicators of wealth and continued awareness of the level of income needed to avoid poverty in retirement.

Annex I: summary of sub-themes: financial circumstances

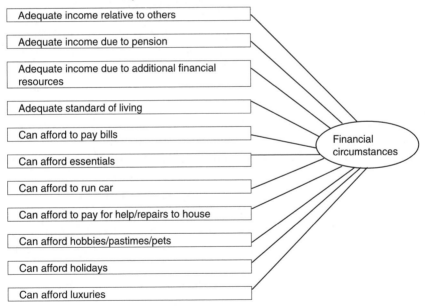

9

Independence and freedom

If I decide I'm going to spend all day in bed and have bacon and eggs at 2 a.m., and go on holiday, or have a new suit, I can do them. Freedom for material things . . . Freedom from pressure.

The freedom to do things when we want to . . . instead of, when you're working, the things you have to do . . . Last week we nipped off for two days to the Lake District, we didn't have to organise time off from work.

Having my health and having a reasonable standard of living. Well they both give you the freedom to do what you want. You are not dependent on anyone.

Doyal and Gough (1991) argued that there are two basic human needs: health and autonomy, which are absolute, not relative to a particular culture. This approach overlaps with Sen's (1992) focus on capabilities, and it could be argued that the achievement of autonomy or capability is essential for individual freedom. There is evidence that lack of autonomy and control over one's life leads to poor health outcomes (Marmot *et al.* 1997; Hemingway and Marmot 1999). In addition, longitudinal data from people aged 70–79 in the MacArthur studies of successful ageing showed that beliefs in one's self-efficacy had a significant impact on perceptions of functional disability, independent of actual underlying physical abilities (Seeman *et al.* 1999).

In retirement, people can be free to indulge in their leisure pursuits, develop new interests and skills, and have the time to do what they want to do; research has shown that people value the freedom of retirement (Crawford 1972). But in practice, retirement can be marred by threats to one's independence, control over life and autonomy (see Box 9.1) from declining health and physical ability, and weak social and economic resources.

The importance of using the coping mechanism of compensatory strategies in the face of life challenges and depleting personal reserves – 'selective optimization with compensation (SOC)' – was emphasized by Baltes and Baltes (1990b). These strategies are expected to enhance one's feelings of

---

Box 9.1 Independence, control and autonomy

- *Independence* is about acting for oneself (e.g. freedom from control in physical functioning, and/or in the ability to organize one's day-to-day life).
- *Perceived self-efficacy and control* over life refers to being able to manage one's life, and its demands, while also being aware that there are areas of life outside one's control.
- *Autonomy* is about being free to make decisions for oneself, free from control by others, and to implement these.

---

self-efficacy and control over life. For example, when selected activities have to be discarded (e.g. due to ill-health or bereavement) strategies need to be activated in order to find new ones and to maximize the chances of maintaining reserves. There is some supportive evidence that these strategies are associated with higher levels of life satisfaction and QoL (Freund and Baltes 1998). However, there are constraints on one's independence and control over one's life imposed by the hierarchical organization of societies.

The whole experience of retirement is partly dependent on income and resources built up over a lifetime, and which are class related (Guillemard 1982; Taylor and Ford 1983). While high levels of perceived self-efficacy are arguably advantageous in the face of life's challenges, it is those in the highest socioeconomic groups who are most endowed with these psychological resources (see Chapter 6). People in low socioeconomic status groups, with lower levels of control over some main areas of their lives (e.g. finances and therefore type of leisure activities, type of occupation and so on), have been reported to be more likely than those in higher status groups to experience low levels of self-esteem and self-efficacy (Blacksher 2002). And it was shown in Chapter 7 that older people who lived in poorer areas, with poor facilities, were the most likely to suffer from barriers to enablement and social engagement, hence restricting their freedom to do what they want, and their independence.

The survey

Ninety-five per cent of respondents to this study had retired from paid work, and in theory were free to pursue their own interests. But this was dependent on their health, the health of close others (e.g. spouses), their personal and neighbourhood social capital, their financial reserves and income and their psychological resources. Some of the pertinent results for health, self-efficacy, personal and neighbourhood social capital and finances are summarized in Boxes 9.2 to 9.6, as they could be hypothesized as enabling factors and, in theory, impact on independence. The fuller results for health and functioning were reported in Chapter 5, self-efficacy in Chapter 6, social capital in Chapter 7 and financial situation in Chapter 8.

In sum, these findings show that the prevalence of long-standing illness was high, although fewer, about a fifth, had great to severe problems with physical functioning. However, sizeable minorities suffered various restrictions on their activities or everyday functioning. Levels of self-efficacy were middle to high for under two-thirds of the sample; most saw relatives or friends at least weekly and about two-thirds were engaged in social activities. About a fifth to a quarter rated their neighbourhoods as poor in provision of facilities for people aged 65+ and for transport. Around a fifth felt crime and safety after dark were issues in their neighbourhoods, and four in ten people never went out after dark. Moreover, a third had no access to a car, and half had an annual income of less than £6240. These are all barriers to independence and control over life in retirement.

Box 9.2 Health

- 62% reported having a long-standing illness, disability or infirmity.
- Of these, 26% said that this condition limited their ability to care for themselves, 42% said it limited their social activities and 37% said it limited them in other ways.
- 46% had slight to moderate difficulties with everyday tasks, and the remaining 22% had great to severe difficulties.

Box 9.3 High self-efficacy

Amount of control over important things in life:

A lot:	44%
Some:	45%
Little or none:	11%

High-middle high scores for self-efficacy (<13) ('EFFIC'): 62%

Box 9.4 Social capital, personal

- 62% (607) saw relatives face to face at least weekly.
- 72% (712) saw friends face to face at least weekly.
- 19% (186) had a high social contact score (frequency of contact with relatives and friends); at the other extreme, 41% (406) had a low score.
- 67% (662) had engaged in 3–12 different social activities over the past month, at the other extreme, 7% (67) had engaged in no activities.

Box 9.5 Social capital, neighbourhood

- 61% scored 'Very good to good' on their overall quality ratings for the facilities in their areas.
- 16% scored as having big problems in their areas overall, and only 4% scored as having no problems.
- 37% regarded their local facilities for people aged 65+ as 'Very good' or 'Good' but, at the other extreme, 21% rated them as 'Very poor' or 'Poor'.
- 47% rated local transport facilities as 'Very good' or 'Good' but, at the other extreme, 20% rated them as 'Very poor' or 'Poor'.
- 24% said that the amount of crime was a 'Very big' or 'Fairly big' problem in their neighbourhood.
- 88% rated their neighbourhoods as 'Very safe' or 'Fairly safe' to walk alone in during the daytime, 6% said it was 'A bit' to 'Very' unsafe and 6% never went out during the daytime.
- 37% rated their neighbourhoods as 'Very safe' or 'Fairly safe' to walk alone in after dark, 21% felt it was 'A bit' to 'Very' unsafe and 42% never went out after dark.

Box 9.6 Financial and living circumstances

- Almost half (47%) were in the lower socioeconomic classes.
- Just over two-thirds (67%) had access to a car or van in the household.
- Almost half (47%) reported having an annual income of less than £6240, just over a fifth (22%) (212) reported having £6240<£9360 and almost a third (31%) (299) reported having between £9360 and £17,680+.

Associations with QoL

Associations with QoL ratings

The associations between the hypothesized enabling characteristics of independence (health, self-efficacy, personal and neighbourhood social capital, socioeconomic factors) and self-rated QoL were reported earlier in Chapters 3 to 8. These will just be summarized here. Health, physical functioning, personal and neighbourhood social capital, but not income or self-efficacy, were all significant, independent predictors of self-rated QoL in the regression model reported in Chapter 3, particularly participation in social activities, frequency of social contacts and safety ratings of the neighbourhood.

Respondents who mentioned their independence as giving their lives quality were more likely to be in the higher social classes, have higher incomes and to have access to a car or van. Consistent with these quantitative results, the analysis of their open-ended and in-depth responses in relation to independence showed that they mainly valued the flexibility, freedom and enjoyment of their lives in retirement, and their access to good transport or to a car, and being able to continue driving, which enabled them to continue to live active lives. Some also mentioned the importance of being able to continue doing things for themselves. And respondents who said their loss of independence took quality away from their lives were more likely than others to have poorer physical functioning and no access to a car or van in the household. Analysis of their open-ended and in-depth responses showed that they also focused on their poor health restricting their activities, and lack of access to transport, which limited their social lives.

While income and other socioeconomic factors were not significant in the regression model of independent predictors of QoL (see Chapter 3), these variables were associated with mention of independence as giving life quality, and having enough money was raised by these respondents as an enabling factor in relation to independence. Having enough money was also mentioned by respondents as one of the main things that gave life quality (see Chapters 3 and 8).

However, while the lay models reported in this chapter emphasize the importance of retaining one's independence in older age, the survey indicator of perceived self-efficacy did not retain statistical significance in the final regression model (see Chapters 3 and 6). It is possible that the measure of self-efficacy was insensitive to issues of independence (as it is really a measure of control), with the implication that, as people themselves say that this area is important for QoL, then improved measures are needed. The effect of self-efficacy on QoL may also have been partly offset by functional status, which did retain significance in the final model (this is supported by the finding from this study that respondents' feelings of having little or no control over the important things in life was independently associated with poor physical functioning) (see Ayis *et al.* 2003). It was also shown in Chapter 6 that self-efficacy was associated with a number of health and social characteristics and appeared to be an enabling characteristic, with mental, physical and social health benefits. Moreover, those in the higher socioeconomic groups had more psychological resources than those in lower social groups.

Lay models

Things that gave life quality

Having and retaining independence was mentioned as an essential feature of a good quality of life by 27% of respondents, particularly being able to do things for oneself, including looking after the home and garden. This was also mentioned by most (69%) of the in-depth interview respondents as giving life quality (see Annex I for a summary of the sub-themes). Men were more likely than women to mention that their independence gave their life quality: 31%:21% respectively. This might reflect the gender differences with functional ability (women had worse functioning, see Chapter 5). However, ability to perform activities of daily living, health status or reported long-standing illness were not associated with mention of independence as giving life quality. There were no associations with mentioning this theme and the age of respondents. Nor were self-efficacy or neighbourhood social capital enabling characteristics associated with mention of independence as giving life quality (e.g. how much control respondents felt they had over the important things in life, overall self-efficacy score, ratings of quality or problems in the area).

So what was mention of independence as giving life quality associated with? Consistent with the perspective that the whole experience of retirement is dependent on income and resources, there were associations with mention of independence as giving life quality and indicators of socioeconomic status. Respondents whose annual income was £9360 and above were more likely to say that independence gave life quality: 33% in comparison with 24% of those with lower incomes. And respondents in the higher social classes I–IIInm were more likely than those in classes IIIm–V to say that independence gave their lives quality: 30%:23% respectively. Just over a third, 34%, of those who said independence gave quality to life had access to a car or van in the household, in comparison with fewer, 11%, who mentioned independence but who had no car access. Access to a car can become important to the retention of independence in the face of declining health and mobility (see p. 195), and was reported in Chapter 6 to be associated with perceived self-efficacy.

The richest source of information about independence *per se*, and insight into the factors affecting it, was obtained from respondents themselves. The information they provided also indicates the type of questions which need to be included in QoL measurement scales, on indicators of independence. Respondents who said that independence gave their lives quality said that they valued their independence, emphasizing that they were still fit enough to retain this. And as one respondent clearly stated, independence and the freedom to do what one wants depends on both health and financial resources:

> Having my health and having a reasonable standard of living. Well they both give you the freedom to do what you want. You are not dependent on anyone.

Consistent with the literature (see Chapter 8), many people who mentioned the theme of independence said they valued the flexibility of being retired, and the lack of time constraints, due to retirement from work, which had previously interfered with their independence. These respondents had a more hedonistic vision of their lives in retirement, and felt they had more time to enjoy life, to see their family and friends and to take up hobbies and new social activities. They were able to 'lie in' in the mornings, to stay up late at night, to eat at more varied times and to take more short breaks away and holidays:

> I've done tremendous long hours of work, in my second job I was in . . . road construction . . . I've done very long hours so . . . my wife and daughter didn't see me all the time and was complaining [*laugh*] that I came in the early hours of the morning [*laugh*] Seven days a week mostly . . . so it wasn't until I retired for them to see a lot of me.

> But . . . we do lay around a lot in bed these days . . . I get up first and get the biscuits and the tea and then we sit there talking. And quite often sometimes we don't come down till about 11, and then, we don't have breakfast, we have brunch then.

Access to a car or good public transport is necessary to enable people to travel more than a short distance away from home. Consistent with the quantitative findings, access to transport played an important role in people's emphasis on their continued independence, especially for those with problems with physical mobility (see also Chapters 6 and 7). Accordingly, a common theme among respondents was that their independence was due to being able to continue driving, and being able to afford to run a car and pay for petrol. This enabled them to travel to places more quickly and comfortably than on public transport, and avoid carrying heavy shopping, especially when they were ill or frail. This recognized need also led to fears about how they would cope if they had to stop driving:

> All we do is shopping, but I mean, I couldn't really put on my husband, because he's had a stroke and two heart attacks, so we couldn't go down the road and carry our shopping home. So we do need transport, although as I say – I have got a son and a daughter that've got cars, but they're working, so . . . you can't sort of, put on them all the time, you can't expect them to do everything for you. You've got to be independent as much as possible. Yeah. So I think, without the car, we'd be pretty stuck.

> At the moment we can drive but I'll be 70 soon and I fear by the time I'm 80 I won't be able to drive and most certainly the quality of life will go down. Everything is dependent on transport and it [public transport] is non-existent at the moment.

> . . . now we have no shops. We don't have a doctor in the village, he's one and a half miles away if I have to walk and I have no motor. My life revolves around a motor. It's a staple of life for me. I run a small motor, [it] doesn't burn much fuel. You can't do anything unless you are mobile. So not being mobile would be a great hindrance.

> The car – it makes my quality of life. It allows me to travel to our caravan, out to get to the seaside . . . I am unable to walk far due to breathing problems and the car gives me independence to get about.

It was reported in Chapter 6 that access to a car or van in the household was associated with greater self-efficacy. Macintyre *et al.* (2000) also reported that access to a car was seen by people as an enabling factor, in terms of giving them greater freedom, life satisfaction, self-esteem, mastery and making them feel safe. Macintyre *et al.* found that people with access to cars reported that they had more freedom than those who usually travelled by public transport. Owner-occupiers with car access had higher levels of mastery, self-esteem, life satisfaction and ontological security (both from the home and from transport) in comparison with those who rented their homes, or those without access to a car.

It was also important to respondents to keep doing as much as they could for themselves, even if they were frail, in order to maintain their self-esteem, ability and interest in life, as well as avoiding dependency:

In the house, doing odd jobs . . . that keeps the interest going and of course the wife always wants this done and that done and I'm capable of doing them in most cases, so I guess that's a hobby in its way . . . mostly the decorating I do myself, but recently when we had the kitchen done up my son-in-law and daughter did all the tiling and all the decorating to save me getting up on the ladder . . . So . . . I like to fiddle around a bit, do things for myself.

(Mr R, in-depth)

I think the most important thing in my life is being able to walk and do my [house] work . . . you know I think that is the main thing. I should hate to have to be in one place all the while. I wouldn't like that . . . that'd be the pits. I would never, never want to do that, because we've never depended on anybody for anything, not even the children.

(Mrs S, in-depth)

The best thing is that I have the health enough to go about and do my own shopping. If you can get on the bus and get about without disturbing anybody else I think that's a big thing really.

It was illustrated in Chapter 7, on social capital, how older people's fears for the future and of losing independence were sometimes heightened when they lived in areas with poor social resources and public services. Access to transport was also said to be important for self-reliance:

If you can get on the bus and get about without disturbing anybody else I think that's a big thing really . . . With the bus pass you can get on and off as you like without paying and saves my legs from walking. I'm happy that I can get about independently, and visit friends and that.

A recurring theme was the value of remaining independent in one's own home; respondents feared loss of independence, autonomy and control over their lives. In societies which value independence, reliance on help may reduce self-esteem and feelings of autonomy. As one woman commented: '[QoL is to] go to town, to go to the library, to be able to control my own affairs, not have to rely on someone else to tell me what to do or if I go out.'

Things that took quality away from life
Just 4% of survey respondents said that loss of their independence (e.g. through declining health, physical mobility or inability to continue driving) made their quality of life bad, although 46% of the in-depth respondents mentioned this. There were no associations with survey respondents' age, sex or socioeconomic indicators (except with access to a car – see p. 197) and

mentioning loss of independence as taking quality away from life. But respondents who had severe or great difficulties with daily living were slightly more likely (11% and 7%, respectively) than those with moderate, slight or no difficulties (2% and 3% respectively) to mention this theme. Similarly, respondents who said they never went out during the day were also more likely than others to mention that loss of independence took quality away from life: 14% and 3% respectively. Those who reported a long-standing illness were slightly more likely than those who did not report this to say that loss of independence took quality away from life: 5% and 2% respectively. This again indicates that, for some, good functional ability was taken for granted until lost. This indicates that people only miss health resources when they no longer have them, and helps to explain the lack of associations between mentioning independence as giving life quality and measures of health and functioning.

In addition, those who said loss of independence took quality away from their lives were slightly less likely to have access to a car or van in the household, although numbers were small: 7% of those who mentioned that loss of independence took quality from life had no access to a car or van, in comparison with fewer, 2%, of those who mentioned this with access.

Poor health was also a main factor blamed by respondents for the loss of their independence, although this was often just one of a series of losses which led some people to lose their confidence and independence. For example, Mrs A had back problems from the physical strain of looking after her ill mother some years before. She now hardly ever went out, and she felt that being isolated indoors most of the time, together with the loss of her husband, had caused her to lose confidence:

> I find I don't have the confidence any more because I'm closed in here. I don't feel secure any more. I'm not sure about anything any more when I go out by myself. I'm not sure I can . . . anymore without my husband. The quality of life . . . I can't walk. If affects my life being stuck in here by myself. And if I have to go somewhere, it's not as if I can go by taxi, and get out of the taxi and go by stick. I don't have the energy . . . I just don't feel like going out any more . . . stuck in here.

Consistent with the quantitative findings, some of those respondents who were unable to drive, who had given up driving due to poor health or the loss of their spouse (who was the driver), or who did not have access to a car, felt that this detracted from their QoL by decreasing their social activities, outings and independence. Sometimes they were reliant on public transport, often with a poor or infrequent service, which again prevented them from travelling, seeing people and doing things they would like to do. One person spoke of being 'marooned'. Widowed women who were unable to drive missed going out in the car with their husbands and pursuing the activities which this enabled them to do. The following examples show how lack of transport meant a reduction in outings and curtailed people's activities:

> I used to play bridge, which I love, but unfortunately I can't go out at night, now, you see, because I haven't a car. But that would improve my quality of life: to be able to play bridge again.
>
> (Mrs C, in-depth)

> R: And another thing that affects my quality of life is that I don't drive. If I had been able to drive and have a car it would have aided my quality of life. Because I would have been able to go easily to see her [her sister]. It's quite complicated by bus because you cannot get a direct bus to C. You've got to change, catch the train then the bus.
> I: How often do you go to see her?
> R: Not often because of that. Sometimes I have a kind friend who takes me there by car.
>
> (Mrs K, in-depth)

> Another thing that I find would improve quality of life, living even here . . . there's no bus service after 6.15 in the evening . . . So in the evening you're really quite cut-off . . . you do find that once winter comes you're completely marooned . . . I mean everyone around here is, we all moan about it [laughs] but there's just no life after, well four in the afternoon in the winter, you've just got the television, and music and that sort of thing [to] amuse yourself . . . [it] is a shame, I think, there aren't more clubs for elderly people to meet perhaps and get together . . . you know . . . companions – you've still got to get to each others' houses, so there is a problem.
>
> (Mrs J, in-depth)

Conclusion

In summary, having and retaining independence was mentioned as an essential feature of a good QoL by 27% respondents, and this was also mentioned by most of the in-depth interview respondents as giving life quality. Independence was said by respondents to be enhanced when they were freed from the constraints placed on them by working hours, if they had retained their health, had an adequate income and could continue to drive/have access to a car. People emphasized the need to be able to do things for oneself, to look after their homes and themselves, to get about and not be dependent on anyone. They disliked being dependent on others for help, even for lifts. Conversely, potential threats to independence and control over one's life included declining health and functioning, poor psychological and social resources, including poor social capital, declining incomes and no access to a car.

The other chapters indicated the importance of these factors to people's QoL. Of course, most respondents could walk and carry out their daily activities with no or few difficulties, but many also reported long-standing illnesses and these were restrictive for a substantial minority. Moreover, almost half of respondents were on extremely low incomes of less than £6240. And, while during the day most respondents appeared to be very active and involved in social activities, after dark this was reversed, with little outside activity taking place. Chapters 3 and 7 emphasized the importance of people feeling safe in their neighbourhoods – and many did not at night. These factors all have implications for public policy.

Annex I: summary of sub-themes: independence

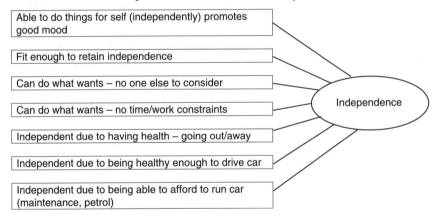

10

Life 18 months later

I will never be an old man. To me, old age is always 15 years older than I am.
Andre B. Buruch; American financier, 1870–1965, www.cyber-nation.com/
victory/quotations/subjects/quotes_ageandaging.html

This chapter focuses on the changes that occur in the lives of older people over a relatively short period, but which can have a major impact on them. Indeed, changes in life, occurring at a greater rate than the perceived average, were associated with decreased morale in the Bonn Longitudinal Study of Ageing (Schmitz-Scherzer and Thomae 1983). As this chapter is concerned with changes over time among an older population group, it also examines attitudes to, and perceptions of, ageing.

Biological ageing can be considered as the progressive constriction of each organ's capacity to maintain homoeostasis when challenged, leading to reduced physiological adaptability, increased susceptibility and vulnerability to disease, and eventually to death (Resnick 1997; Troen 2003). However, as indicated in Chapter 1, there appears to be some plasticity of the ageing processes, including in late old age, and it has been suggested that theories of homeostasis require modification. For example, evidence on ageing and risk of cognitive impairment shows that, despite strong relationships with chronological age, this impairment is not inevitable (Grundy 2001). There is evidence of beneficial results for mental health of continued mental stimulation in older age (Khaw 1997). Furthermore, experimental studies have demonstrated that deterioration in muscle strength associated with ageing is reversible (McMurdo 2000; Greig 2002; Malbut et al. 2002). Large numbers of very old people have reported that they feel relatively healthy (Nybo et al. 2001), although the 'oldest old' (e.g. those aged 85+) have also been reported to have lower levels of well-being, and satisfaction with life than those of younger ages (Bowling et al. 1991, 1999). However, the results of the QoL survey reported in this book support the relative physical, psychological and social health of most people aged 65 and over, and their perceptions of having a good QoL. But, of course, there was also diversity among respondents, and wide individual variations in maintaining health, functioning and independence. A person with reduced functional capacity, social and psychological resources is likely to have more difficulty retaining independence when faced with disease than another of the same chronological age with greater reserve capacity. Indeed, commonly cited risk factors for the negative events in older age (e.g. entry into institutional care) include not just functional and cognitive ability, chronic disease and co-morbidities, but social isolation and absence of social support (see review by Bowling 1994).

Chronological age is only one of the factors which influence the process of ageing. This indicates that, given the wide variations between individuals in this process, it is more logical to examine patterns of ageing instead of statistical norms. Indicators of functional and subjective age would be of value in research, as supplements to chronological age, if they could tap the cumulative gains and losses in capacity amassed throughout life. Research on subjective age, or age identity, has indicated that people who feel younger than their years rate their health, satisfaction with life and QoL as higher than other people (Mutran and Burke 1979; Barak and Schiffman 1981; Steitz and McClary 1988; Logan *et al.* 1992; Grundy and Bowling 1999; Michalos and Zumbo 2000; Michalos *et al.* 2001). Staats *et al.*(1993) found that those older people who identified their social activities as belonging to an age group younger than their own were also more likely to report a higher QoL. Age identity is worthy of further exploration as a potentially more sensitive indicator than chronological age in research on ageing. For example, it has been reported to be a better predictor of mortality than chronological age or health status (Carp and Carp 1981; Markides and Pappas 1982).

The follow-up study

Ageing is dynamic, and should not be regarded as a static entity, observed at a single point in time (Bryant *et al.* 2001). The aim of the follow-up survey questionnaire, then, was to elicit changes in people's QoL, as well as attitudes to ageing and subjective age (or age identity: how old people feel) (see Chapter 2 for details of questions). Given reported associations in the literature between QoL and how old one feels, the analyses also aimed to investigate predictors of subjective age, defined in terms of how old people actually feel in relation to their actual age. The data has been presented more fully elsewhere (Bowling *et al.* 2005). These results are reported here in two sections.

As was pointed out in Chapter 2, out of the 999 baseline survey respondents, 786 (79%) agreed to be recontacted. At approximately 18 months after their baseline survey interview, these respondents were followed up with a postal questionnaire. Over two-thirds, 68% (533), of those sent a postal questionnaire returned it completed. In addition, the in-depth interviews with a small sub-sample were repeated. This chapter focuses on the results of the postal survey. Some of the in-depth interview material is used to illustrate changes in QoL.

Changes since baseline interview

Changes in life and health

Older age is often a time of increasing challenges to a person's physical and mental health, and to emotional and social well-being. In reply to an open-ended question about the main changes in their lives – good and bad – in the last six months, almost four in ten people, 38%, reported a major change in their lives over this relatively short time period. Consistent with the deterioration in ADL score for about a quarter of respondents, most of these reported deteriorating health and functioning:

◆ 60% reported that their health and sensory functions had deteriorated;

◆ 15% reported another person's health had worsened;

◆ 9% had been bereaved;

◆ 6% said they were less functionally able or less able to get out and about;

◆ 6% reported stopping social activities.

Few respondents reported good changes, but the most common of these were moving home, usually nearer family or family moving closer to them (8%), improved health (5%), becoming a grandparent (4%) and improving financial investments (4%).

Changes in QoL since baseline interview

For most respondents, QoL self-ratings had stayed the same (52%) or improved (15%) since baseline, although for a third, 33%, QoL ratings had deteriorated. It is unknown to what extent these results may be partly due to response shift (Sprangers and Schwartz 1999). Significant changes were also detected in physical functioning (ADL/IADL score) at follow-up survey. In support of this, the repeated in-depth interviews at 12 months post-baseline also suggested that changes in functional ability were responsible for people rating their QoL as worse. Physical functioning scores had deteriorated for just over a quarter of respondents, 26%, it was unchanged for almost two-thirds, 63%, and had improved for just 11%. However, there were no significant changes in reported health status or long-standing illness, suggesting that the ADL items were more sensitive to change.

It was hypothesized that baseline indicators of better physical health and functioning, higher levels of social activity, help, support, good mental health and psychological resources would be associated with positive self-rated QoL at follow-up. The justification for this was an expectation of i) the continuation of the enabling features of health and functioning reported at baseline, and ii) the continuing protective effects of good social and psychological resources reported at baseline.

At the bivariate level of analysis, neither sociodemographic or socioeconomic variables, nor baseline physical health or functional status, were associated with changes in QoL at 18 months. Changes in QoL ratings between surveys were associated just with selected baseline psychological and social measures: self-efficacy, anxiety and depression (GHQ score), number of social activities that respondents were engaged in, number of areas of life they received practical help with, and emotional support in. These variables were associated with changes in QoL scores between surveys in the expected directions (see Box 10.1). Thus baseline low self-efficacy, poor psychological health, having no or fewer than five different social activities, and lower levels of help and support were associated with a deterioration in QoL ratings at follow-up. These data are supportive of social and psychological theories, which emphasize the need to build up one's social and psychological resources over time. This is in order to enhance one's reserves of these in older age, when they can be deployed to enhance coping in the face of life challenges (see Chapter 1).

A hierarchical multiple linear regression was used to explore the independent predictive ability of these baseline co-variates on QoL score at follow-up (dependent variable). Health and functional status were also entered into the model, despite their non-significance at bivariate level, as they were considered as *a priori* hypotheses, on the basis of the literature, the baseline data and lay reports (see Chapters 1, 3 and 5). Baseline QoL score was entered as the first predictor examined followed, in subsequent steps, by these other variables. This procedure is known as residualized change analysis, and provides an estimation of the effects of the independent variables on changes in self-rated QoL between assessments (George *et al.* 1989).

Box 10.1 Baseline associations with a worse QoL score at follow-up

◆ Those with the worst self-efficacy scores (15 – 23) at baseline were more likely than others to have a worse QoL score at follow-up: 49% compared with
32% of middle scoring groups and 25% of the highest scoring group for self-
efficacy.

◆ Those who scored as anxious/depressed at baseline were more likely than
non-cases to have a worse QoL score at follow-up: 44% compared with 30%
of non-cases.

◆ Those with less than five different social activities in the past month at baseline were more likely than those with more activities to have a worse QoL
score at follow-up: 41% (9) of those with no social activities and 40% of
those with between one and four activities had a worse QoL score, compared with fewer, 23%, of those with five to twelve activities.

◆ Those who had least help (with a lift, help when ill, money, errands) and
support in a personal crisis were slightly more likely than those who had
most help and support to have a worse QoL score at follow-up: 29% of those
with help with one to three areas had a worse QoL score compared with
33% of those who had help in four to five areas.

Each entered variable achieved statistical significance in the model, except
number of areas helped and supported in. The greatest predictor of QoL score
at follow-up was QoL score at baseline, which accounted for most of the variation between groups: the adjusted R^2 was 26.7%. Number of social activities
explained a further 2.5% of the variance, although adding in number of areas
helped and supported in explained no more. Adding in self-efficacy explained a
further 1.5%, and adding in GHQ score also explained a further 1.5%. Adding in
health and physical functioning explianed another 4.1% of the variance. The
total of explained variance was 36.3% (adjusted R^2), and the final model was
highly significant (F: $p<0.001$). These results give most support to the importance of having good health and functioning and some, although more limited,
support to theories about the importance of social participation and psychological resources for coping effectively with the challenges of later life. Future follow-
ups of the sample can provide more detailed information for further modelling.

Lay models

The in-depth follow-up interviews provided more insightful and dynamic
information about why people felt their QoL had changed. People attributed

decreases in their QoL to deteriorating health, which limited the things they wanted to do, and to the worsening health of a spouse, which required them to spend more time caring for them and also led to greater anxiety. Some people said their QoL was worse due to loss of family members and/or friends through death. Better psychological well-being, slightly improved finances due to pension increases, improvements to their home (decorating, new furniture) and increases in social activity were attributed to increases in QoL.

Deteriorating health, their own or that of a close other's, was mentioned by most of these respondents as the domain that had changed one year later. A deterioration in their spouse's health could detract from their own QoL due to greater worry, having to carry out more household tasks, spending more time caring for them, and not being able to go away. Mr E and Mr F gave examples of the impact of their spouse's health, and their own, on their lives (see Cases 10.1 and 10.2).

Mrs V gave another example of how worsening health led to worsening QoL. Her quality of life ratings had deteriorated between interviews from 'Very good' to being described as 'useless'. This was due to a decline in health preventing her from doing many of the things that she wanted to do. She could no longer garden and found it more difficult to walk:

Well actually there has been quite a lot of change. Quality of life is useless. Which I presume is to do with the leukaemia. I've had two lots of treatment, tablets. There's no cure for it, it's just trying to make my quality of life better. Which the first lot did, I was quite . . . I had about ten days when I felt quite perky. You know, went for a nice walk and I was eating much better. And then I started to go downhill again and they gave me another course of tablets and unfortunately they didn't do any good at all . . . I've been dreadful. In fact . . . since Sunday, I've been able to keep food down, prior to that I was just vomiting everything up, sleeping all day, it's as much as I can do to walk up the garden. I certainly can't push the vacuum cleaner, my husband has to do all that, and the cooking and such like . . . it's just one of them things you've got to accept, and that's it. I just want to be [well] for a month's time, because my first, eldest grand-daughter's getting married . . . Well, you know, I don't want to spoil her day by not being able to go.

Some respondents said their lives were worse due to their poorer mental health, which was usually said to be due to declining physical health, their role as carer, and to the loss of friends or family members (see Case 10.3).

Case 10.1 Mr E

At baseline interview, Mr E described how good his QoL could have been if his wife had not suffered from Alzheimer's disease:

> . . . in my particular case, my quality of life has been completely altered by the fact that my wife suffers from Alzheimer's disease . . . you will enjoy a good quality of life if you could go abroad . . . if you liked . . . if you could buy what you desired without worrying too much about where the money was coming from, and in all these cases, I would have score[d] highly . . . till my wife suffered from Alzheimer's.

Mr E spoke about the strain of caring for his wife, because she undid the things he achieved, such as housework:

> . . . my quality of life is overwhelmingly . . . altered, and focused by my wife's . . . problems . . . I've often thought I look after three people. My wife used to look after me, she used to feed me, she used to do my laundry . . . If I was ill she'd nurse me . . . She'd make sure my tie was on straight . . . that kind of thing, and now I have to do all that for myself . . . I do everything for her; she does nothing. I do the washing up, the laundry, the ironing, the dusting . . . the vacuum cleaning, all the financial stuff, she doesn't know what money is . . . so I look after two people, really I didn't look after anyone before . . . I did my job . . . I didn't have to think about who was going to press me trousers or who was going to wash me shirt, I did none of those – well now I do it all, and I do it all for her. And then there is a third person, a third person undoes all I do, the third person hides me keys, the third person floods the kitchen by leaving the taps on in the bathroom, err, the third person hides my letters . . . it's all stress and strain. And of course that very much affects my quality of life.

At his follow-up interview, Mr E felt that his QoL had declined further because of his wife's worsening health. She had become incontinent and was less mobile, and required more physical care. Paradoxically, Mr E described how his caring responsibilities were easier as his wife would sit still for longer periods, and would no longer undo the things he achieved. However, Mr E felt more upset as it was now clear to him that his wife would not be able to live at home for much longer. Due to another year of stress, Mr E felt that overall his QoL had worsened:

> Well, it's [QoL] gone down because it's another year, you know, it's, I suppose it's another 12 months of extra, what, nervous tension, whatever you like to call it . . .

Case 10.2 Mr F

At his baseline interview, Mr F, aged 76, was living with his second wife. Mr F spoke of how worrying about his wife's health adversely affected his own. A year later, he said that his QoL had worsened. He had been diagnosed with an irregular heartbeat, he suffered from breathlessness and poor eyesight, and as a result there were some activities which he was no longer able to do:

> ... things are not the same, if I can sort of remember back ... when nothing was wrong with you at all, when ... you could get out and wash the car when you wanted to ... We've got a lot of shrubs round the garden, I used to cut them two or three times a year ... with ... just ordinary trimmers, I'm not sure how far I'd get with them now. And one other thing that does bother me is, is climbing. Getting onto steps ... and things like that. Because I do notice I get a little giddy lately ... But another thing ... I can't cut my own toenails any more ... because ... my toenails got so hard now, and the eyesight I can't ... see them obviously ... And ... her [wife's] wrists are not strong enough even to try and help ... I'm sure she would if she could, but she can't do it. So ... that's another job I got for ... the health centre.

Mr F had also stopped driving long distance, which meant that he was unable to see his children as regularly. He said he had adjusted to these problems using a strategy of acceptance, keeping busy and using downward comparisons:

> ... I sit down sometimes and think ... is there any part of me that's working properly ... as time goes on, one [health problem] develops sooner, then another starts, and ... the only thing that keeps it going ... is [accepting it and] to think that there's a lot of people worse off than you are ... And then when you get this thing and it's ... long-term ... and that sort of makes you fed up, you think oh ... it means it's here forever ... you think you're going to live with it for the rest of your life. And ... that knocks you back a bit. For a while, until you kind of accept it ... It's very difficult to accept that you've got a complaint but then once you've accepted it ... you can actually live with it.
>
> I: But how did you ... come to accept it?
>
> R: ... you help yourself by thinking about others really. You kind of think you've got the worst complaint on this earth. But then you've got to find something to ... kind of buck you up again, got to find something, got to think about something, take your mind off what you're doing and what's wrong with you and try and think about something else. And I think it'll always work, providing that you've got the will-power.

Case 10.3 Mr L

Mr L was a widower living by himself. He provides an example of how the onset of depression detracted from his QoL because he had 'given up caring' about things such as his appearance and the upkeep of his home. His depression appeared to have been triggered by his worsening health, and the deaths of close friends since his first interview.

He rated his QoL as 'good' at his baseline interview. The factors he said gave his life quality then were being financially comfortable and having close relationships with his family. He did voluntary work, but also said that he was lonely and craved more company, saying that voluntary work was not the same as socializing. He had a fairly pessimistic outlook on life and he tended to focus on negative events which might occur in the future.

One year on, Mr L's QoL had changed for the worse. His health had declined for he had been suffering from chesty colds and difficulty breathing, and his memory had deteriorated, but these problems remained undiagnosed. It also took him a long time to get up in the morning and he had difficulty walking, which had restricted his social and other activities:

> That is terrible. People don't understand it, you see. It takes me three hours to get up, before I'm ready to go out . . . I say to myself 'I must try to do it quicker' but I cannot. And sometimes I've got to go out for somewhere at 9 a.m., and that means I have to get up at 6 a.m. to get out. It's hard work and I'm worn out . . . short of breath . . . you should try walking down the shops with me . . . sometimes I only get half way, if it's a bad day . . . I don't go anywhere.

More striking was a change in his attitude, towards boredom and despondency. This was mainly apparent from an altered approach to his appearance and the upkeep of his house:

> . . . the decision I've made is that I couldn't care less any more, that's the state I'm in at the moment . . . I used to dress up and make myself decent, always wore a collar and tie. I couldn't care less what I looked like now.
> I: Has that changed in the last year?
> R: Yes, that's changed, you can see me now in pullovers and things, not my suit. Only when I have meetings, special meeting, but I just don't care anymore. And I don't care about this place, I've let it go, since you came here I've done nothing to it. I couldn't care less. I only get the Hoover out once every couple of months . . .

In the period between his baseline and follow-up interviews, Mr L had lost several friends, including a very close friend. Their deaths upset him, and he felt that they contributed to his negative attitude:

> ... the other most distressing thing is I've lost so many friends ... That's very distressing because I've lost some of my best friends and we've had deaths in the family too ... And that doesn't help your morale I can tell you, it's very distressing ... and ... I couldn't care less any more. And that's been the biggest change in my attitude since last time. I don't care what I look like when I go out, whether this place goes to pot, I couldn't care less.
>
> I: Why do you think that's come about?
>
> R: It's probably because it's been a bad year, and I lost so many of my good friends, and I have to go to funerals which is very depressing ... I suppose it's one thing after the other, and you think 'How long have I got?' All these things add up.

Loss of social relationships, leading to loss of social activities and outings, was commonly mentioned as leading to a worse QoL:

> So that's another friend ... that I used to see and go places with occasionally. Now that's the trouble you see, as you get older, you keep losing friends, and the older you are you end up with ... you've lost all your friends. I've lost all my relatives of my own generation now, my brother was the last one. And I've only got my niece and my nephew now so, they're coming up to retirement. My nephew retires this Christmas. But they live in H so I don't see a great deal of them.

> I lost ... friends and it makes a kind of hole in your life. And, you know, you miss them because you went on holiday, or there's one I used to meet regularly in Edinburgh and go out for a meal, things like that.

However, others said they felt their QoL had improved since their baseline interview due to now being able to cope with earlier bereavement, and said they had deliberately made use of coping strategies, such as acceptance or feeling lucky to be alive:

> ... when you get on a bit in life you accept it ... I'm still alive, I'm lucky, they've ... gone. And especially ones that were very old, you, you're very happy that they have gone, because ... they were suffering. So I just take it as the way of life, or death ... And just think I'm one of the lucky ones. I think there's no good getting cross about these things. If it's going to happen it's going to happen. And everyone's got to go sooner or later ... And people do say, 'I know you must know what I'm going through' sort of thing ... my philosophy is, don't feel sorry for yourself when you lose someone near to you, you're the lucky one that's still alive.

209

Similarly, Mrs I had been widowed a few months before her baseline interview. A year after her interview, Mrs I's life had improved considerably. She said she felt better about her husband's death, feeling that she had been in a daze during the period of her initial interview. It was only recently that she had begun to feel more in control of her life again. She spoke of wanting to lead a more active life, for example by getting a passport and going away somewhere:

> . . . the year before last was the dramatic change in life, but the last year it has been coming back from that, you know, building up a new lifestyle, a new kind of life. Um [*pause*] sometimes I think I don't remember much of last year. I think I existed getting up, looking after [my grand-daughter], getting back, going to bed and that was it. Still trying to go out a couple nights a week . . . but I didn't want to go very far. I was feeling that I wanted to stay around here for some reason. But that's beginning to go now, I'm beginning to want to get up and out and do things . . . I can deal with things better. Before I felt I was just [not] myself for a wee while. I think possibly I decided I would let myself go down and then come back up from there. But . . . I always went out and things. As I say, I feel now I would like to get my passport, that kind of thing . . . book a holiday somewhere, things like that. So I would say that the grieving process is coming. They say you never forget, but you begin to live with it. You get used to living on your own.

These examples show the knock-on effects of various life events which affect QoL. For example, respondents reported that it is not bad health *per se* that caused them to rate their QoL as poor, but rather its negative impact on their ability to socialize or look after their homes. However, the examples presented here also demonstrate the strength and resilience of older people, in the face of accumulating life events.

Attitudes to ageing

At postal follow-up survey, in response to an open-ended question, the most commonly listed *best things* about growing older related to independence and freedom, the slower pace of life and more time:

- independence and freedom; doing things one wants to; pleasing oneself; freedom from time constraints (32%);

- slower pace of life (24%);

- more time to pursue own interests/hobbies (21%);

- more time for family and friends (15%);

- having more knowledge about life (13%);

- being able to enjoy grandchildren without having to look after them (13%);

- going away on holidays (8%);

- not having a mortgage/debts/not paying tax/being financially secure/being able to spend money on oneself (8%).

Most responses to an open-ended question on the *worst things* about growing older related to worsening health, loss of independence, and, for a few, fear of death:

- poor health and deteriorating senses (52%);

- loss of independence due to deteriorating health and functioning and being unable to do what one wants (from getting out and about to going on holiday) (40%);

- fear of dying and not knowing how long they had left to live (12%);

- loneliness (7%);

- having insufficient money; increasing costs of living (6%).

Similarly, the most commonly mentioned *fears* about growing older, which respondents listed, related to ill-health and dependency:

- ill-health and deteriorating physical ability (38%);

- physical dependency (33%);

- entering residential or nursing home care (12%);

- being alone/not having anyone to help or care for one (12%);

- being a burden on others (8%);

- lack of money/debts (5%);

- dying and leaving their partner/children (5%).

As with definitions of QoL, then, having independence and freedom, avoiding dependency, ill-health and loss of functioning were important concerns here.

Subjective age

Respondents were asked how old they felt in comparison with their actual age. Over half felt considerably younger than their actual ages (see Table 10.1).

Over half of respondents believed that old age started at age 80 or more. Just 10% said they felt old age commenced before the age of 70, 17% said it began at

Table 10.1 How old respondents felt compared with actual age

How old (*n* = 533)?	%	(*n*)
Up to 10 years younger than their age	13	(72)
Between 10<25 years younger	31	(163)
More than 25 years younger	6	(32)
Younger, unspecified how much	6	(32)
Same age	38	(204)
Older	6	(29)

70<75, and 21% said it began at 75<80, while 31% believed it started at ages 80<85 and 21% at 85+. When they considered someone to be old was associated with their own age – the older they were, the later old age was said to commence. For example, over two-thirds, 69%, of those aged 65<70 said old age commenced at age 75+, rather than at a younger age, in comparison with over three-quarters, 78%, of those aged 75+. This is consistent with other research among the general public of all ages in England (Age Concern England 1992) and is in line with the folk wisdom, 'You are as young as you feel'.

There were no consistent or significant trends with actual, chronological age of respondents and the subjective age they felt, indicating that self-perceived age is independent of chronological age. And whether respondents felt younger, the same or older than their actual age was not associated with respondents' sex. Nor was it associated with their familial longevity (ages of live/at death of parents, same-sex siblings).

In marked contrast to subjective age, there were no differences by respondents' real chronological age and their social characteristics and circumstances, psychological attitudes or reported health status, although those aged over 75 did have worse physical functioning. The subjective age that respondents actually felt was a more sensitive indicator than chronological age in relation to these variables. The results are summarized in Box 10.2.

The association of socioeconomic status with subjective age again suggests the pervasive effects of social structure on perceptions (and see Chapter 6), although this did not retain significance in the further modelling.

Modelling, using hierarchical multiple linear regression, was used to explore the independent predictive ability of these co-variates on age identity (dependent variable). Subjective age identity was a (continuous) variable

---

Box 10.2 Associations with subjective age

Respondents who felt younger than their years were more likely than those who felt the same, or older to:

◆ have better baseline mental health (GHQ score) (15%, 26%, 40% respectively);
◆ have better baseline health status (49% rated their health as 'Excellent' or 'Very good' in comparison with 34% and 3% respectively);
◆ have better physical functioning (ADL/IADL score) at baseline (44% had no problems with functioning compared with 25% and 0% respectively);
◆ have unchanged physical functioning, rather than deteriorated, at follow-up: 71%, 54%, 64% respectively remained the same;
◆ feel a high sense of mastery and control over their life (self-efficacy) at baseline: 30%, 21% and 23% respectively scored highest in self-efficacy;
◆ report having more (5+) social activities at baseline: 54%, 31%, 10% respectively;
◆ rate their baseline quality of life more positively: 64%, 41%, 45% respectively;
◆ report unchanged (as opposed to deteriorated) QoL at follow-up: 61%, 45%, 19% respectively;
◆ be in higher socioeconomic groups (64%, 48%, 47% respectively were in the higher social classes I–IIInm, old coding);
◆ be more educated: 40%, 27%, 26% had 'O level' equivalent or above;
◆ be home owners: 88%, compared with 76% and 67% respectively.

---

measuring how many years older or younger than their actual age respondents felt (a score of '0' represented feeling the same as one's actual age). The final regression model showed that baseline physical health and functional status, and reported changes in these at follow-up, explained 20.4% of the variance in self-perceived age ratings. Adding baseline psychological morbidity (anxiety/depression), feelings and fears about ageing at follow-up explained just a further 0.8% of the variance, making the total variance explained 21.2%. Socioeconomic indicators lost significance in earlier models and were not included in the final model. Although the greatest part of the variance remains unexplained, the implication is that good health and functioning are still the main independent predictors of feeling younger than one's years, followed by lack of psychological morbidity and positive attitudes towards ageing (see Bowling *et al.* 2005 for detailed analysis).

These results support other research which has reported that people who feel younger than their years report better physical and mental health status, and rate their satisfaction with aspects of their lives, or QoL, as higher (Mutran and Burke 1979; Barak and Schiffman 1981; Steitz and McClary 1988; Logan *et al.* 1992; Grundy and Bowling 1999; Michalos and Zumbo 2000; Michalos *et al.* 2001). It is possible that future cohorts of people in their 60s and beyond will be even more reluctant to perceive themselves as 'old'. Indeed, there is some evidence from the UK that people in their 50s share similar attributes and behaviours to people in their 30s and 40s than with people older than themselves (Scales and Scase 2000). This is of importance in relation to health policy and prediction of trends.

Conclusion

While most respondents' QoL ratings were unchanged, or improved between surveys, six in ten people reported deteriorations in their health and senses; ADL scores had deteriorated for just over a quarter, although they were unchanged for almost two-thirds. The results of the regression analyses gave most support to the importance of having good health and functioning for maintaining or improving QoL over time. However, the follow-up period was relatively short (about 18 months). Future follow-ups of the sample will provide more detailed information for further modelling.

The best things about ageing were said to be about independence, having time to enjoy life and freedom. But enjoyment of ageing depends on having a wide range of resources, not just psychological resources – for example, reserves of finances, social support, neighbourhood social capital and health. The worse things about ageing, and fears about ageing, related to people's worsening health, decreasing independence and fear of dependency – which threatened independence, freedom and social participation. This chapter has illustrated how life events, particularly poor health and bereavement, can have knock-on effects on people's lives. As with definitions of QoL (see Chapters 3, 5 and 9), having independence and freedom, and having one's health and functional ability, were main themes, illustrating their importance to older people.

In contrast to earlier disengagement theories of ageing, the results presented here also showed that most respondents felt considerably younger than their actual ages, and subjective age was not associated with actual, chronological age. The older the respondent, then the later old age was said to commence. Age was a more sensitive indicator of health and functioning and psychological outlook, for example, than chronological age. Consistent with the literature on age identity, or subjective age, people who felt younger than their years were also more likely, at baseline, to be in better health and, to a lesser extent, have more social and psychological resources.

The results indicate that social structures within society that are based on rigid age cut-offs (e.g. conventional retirement ages of 65) require urgent rethinking. And, given the relative insensitivity of chronological age reported here, measurement of non-chronological age also requires development, and can be used to supplement chronological age in social, psychological, medical and epidemiological research. Fennel *et al.* (1988) cited J.B. Priestley's reply, on the publication of his 99th book at the age of 79, to the question 'What was it like to be old?'. His response makes a fitting conclusion to this chapter:

> It was as though walking down Shaftesbury Avenue as a fairly young man, I was suddenly kidnapped, rushed into a theatre and made to don the grey hair, the wrinkles and other attributes of age, then wheeled on-stage. Behind the appearance of age I am the same person, with the same thoughts, as when I was younger.
> (reported by Puner 1974: 7. Reproduced with permission of Palgrave Macmillan)

11

Discussion: implications for ageing well in the twenty-first century

Grow old with me!

The best is yet to be,

(Browning [1864] 1979)

Perls and Silver (1999) stated that living to 100 has become a new social phenomenon. They cited data from the Terman Longitudinal study (in which gifted Californian schoolchildren were followed up for more than 70 years), which showed that key factors in achieving very old age were remaining disease-free, preserving cognitive abilities, maintaining preventive (healthy) lifestyles, having stress resistant personalities, being immune to neuroticism and also genetic factors.

The research focus is also increasingly on how to promote 'active ageing' and the enhancement of QoL in older age. Although evidence is still being accumulated, it has been argued that 50% of the ageing process is influenced by one's DNA, but the other 50% can also be influenced (www.anti-age.org.uk). Gingold (1999) argued that disease prevention is an integral part of influencing successful ageing, and that with this comes improved health and fitness which influence independence, continued social participation and involvement with life, feelings of well-being, self-esteem and satisfaction with life. Conventional advice for maintaining health in older age includes taking more exercise, giving up smoking, eating more fruit and vegetables, keeping socially and mentally active and drinking more water (Research into Ageing 2004), as well as many calls for strategies to prevent chronic illness, to enhance cognitive performance and physical functioning, to promote mental and physical health and to improve social skills.

Evidence from the social sciences suggests that more is needed, including promoting an individual's self-efficacy, a positive disposition and a tendency to make downward social comparisons to make oneself feel better about one's position in life. One of the main psychological strategies proposed for maintaining well-being and promoting self-mastery in older age is the use of self-enhancing social comparisons (Ryff 1999). But social comparisons are just one of several ways in which people may cope with problems, construct and evaluate the gap between desired and achieved reality (Sherif 1936; Hyman 1942; Festinger 1954), and offset the effects of adverse events and circumstances. Self-efficacy, in particular, has also been held to be an important factor in the promotion of mental health and QoL of older people in their adaptation to the challenges of ageing and ageing well (Baltes and Baltes 1990a, 1990b; Blazer 2002). In addition, as pointed out in Chapter 4, the largest body of empirical research on the predictors of well-being has focused on the structure, functioning and supportiveness of human relationships, the social context in which people live and their integration within society. While there is some supportive evidence of these links, they are not as strong predictors of well-being as physical health and functioning.

Are these sufficient for enhancing QoL in older age? Despite early research by social gerontologists on constituents of QoL, the factors which influence QoL in older age have remained largely theoretical. Doubt has even been raised about whether such a complex construct can be defined and measured at all. However, results from the survey of people aged 65 and over living at home in Britain, which are presented here, indicate that older people were able to define what is good and bad QoL, and to suggest ways in which this could be enhanced both for themselves and for other people their age.

Summary of main findings

The results of this research indicate that, in general, life in older age can be described positively for most people, with the majority reporting their QoL to be good, and, for most, these ratings were unchanged, or had improved, at follow-up. Most respondents also rated their mental and physical health positively, were actively engaged in social activities and felt supported. At follow-up, the main change mentioned by respondents was their declining health. They also reported many good things that they enjoyed about growing older, including their independence and freedom, although the worst things about growing older included worsening health and consequent loss of independence.

Comparisons of the results with the author's earlier work indicates that older and younger adults' general perspectives of QoL are similar (Bowling 1995a, 1995b, 1996), but older people simply have more life challenges (e.g. risk of declining health, bereavement, loss of mobility, reduced income) which affect their priorities. As some respondents indicated, they felt like young people inside. Also consistent with this earlier research, men and women, and people in different older age groups emphasized different themes, in reflection of their traditional roles in life and differing priorities.

The main independent indicators of self-rated good QoL at baseline in the regression model, and which explained 26.70% of the variance in QoL ratings (which is sizeable on subjective topics) were: making (downward) social comparisons between oneself and others who were worse-off; having an optimistic outlook; having good health and physical functioning; having more social activities, frequent social contacts and support; not feeling lonely; having good local facilities; and feeling safe in one's area of residence (see Box 11.1 for summary).

These factors contributed more to perceived QoL than objective socioeconomic indicators such as education, social class, income or home ownership. This supports earlier research showing that subjective indicators were more predictive than objective socioeconomic indicators of self-rated QoL (Zizzi *et al.* 1998; Bowling and Windsor 2001).

Box 11.1 Summary of the regression modelling

The main, independent predictors of self-rated QoL in the regression model were:

♦ people's standards of social comparison and expectations in life – making downward social comparisons with those worse off;
♦ a sense of optimism and belief that 'all will be well in the end' rather than a tendency to think the worst;
♦ having good health and physical functioning;
♦ engaging in a large number of social activities, frequent social contacts, feeling helped and supported, not feeling lonely;
● living in a neighbourhood with good community facilities and services, including transport;
● feeling safe in one's neighbourhood;
● self-efficacy, and having a sense of control over one's life, lost significance in the model, but was possibly a mediating variable.

Box 11.2 Lay models of quality of life identified by the open-ended survey questions and in-depth interviews

Older people's views of quality of life were:

- having good social relationships with family, friends and neighbours;
- participating in social and voluntary activities, and individual interests;
- having good health and functional ability;
- living in a good home and neighbourhood;
- having a positive outlook and psychological well-being;
- having an adequate income;
- maintaining independence and control over one's life.

The main lay themes, which people believed formed the foundations for a good QoL, which emerged from both the open-ended survey responses and the in-depth, follow-up interviews, overlapped considerably. They supported the results of the regression model, but with the addition of two other key factors: the importance of the perception of having an adequate income, and of retaining independence and control over one's life. The key determinants of QoL which emerged from both of these interview methods are shown in Box 11.2.

All respondents expressed a wide range of more personal reasons about why the QoL themes they mentioned were important to them. Each set of the lay themes, which were derived from the two different methods used, overlapped considerably. The main difference was that the in-depth interview approach allowed ample time to explore QoL and so most themes were mentioned by most respondents. This was in contrast to the semi-structured interviews, which imposed greater time constraints on the interview due to the length of the questionnaire, and thus people mentioned fewer themes each. Hence, although there was the danger of bias from response shift between the two interviews (adjustment of expectations over time, leading to different ratings of life), which could have affected the comparisons between the datasets, this did not appear to have been over-influential in this study. In sum, the comparison of results from the triangulated approach indicated that overall QoL is built on a series of interrelated drivers (main themes), while individuals may emphasize varying constituent parts (sub-themes).

The results of the quantitative analyses, then, were remarkably consistent with lay views. But the exceptions were that both income and perceived self-efficacy lost statistical significance in the regression model, which assessed independent predictors of QoL. In contrast, these aspects of life (having enough money, retaining independence and control) were emphasized as important in the lay models derived from both the in-depth and semi-structured interviews. The implication is that, as people themselves say that these areas are important for QoL, better indicators of them are needed, and they need encompassing within a model of QoL.

Self-efficacy is a theoretically important concept in this context (Baltes and Baltes 1990b; Blazer 2002), and was found to be associated with better psychological and physical health and social resources. However, it was influenced by socioeconomic position, suggesting there were social structure barriers to its development. It is possible that the measure of self-efficacy was mediating between variables in the regression model of QoL. For example, the effect of self-efficacy on QoL may have been partly mediated by functional status which did retain significance in the final model. Improved measurement, relevant to older people, is probably required – the measure of self-efficacy used was not designed specifically for use with older people. And, in relation to income, it is possible that in older age, when incomes are more levelled due to people's reliance mainly on pensions (although a wide range of annual income still exists), objective indicators of financial status are less sensitive than perceived financial circumstances. This finding has implications for the design of measurement instruments (i.e. it is important to tap perceptions).

Combining both the quantitative and more qualitative approaches, then, this study suggests that the main building blocks, or drivers, of QoL in older age can be summarized as follows:

- having an optimistic outlook and psychological well-being, especially in relation to making downward rather than unrealistic upward social comparisons;

- having good health and physical functioning;

- having good social relationships, preventing loneliness, and feeling helped and supported;

- maintaining social roles, especially engaging in a large number of social activities, including voluntary work, and having individual interests;

- living in a neighbourhood with good community facilities and services, including access to affordable transport, and feeling safe in one's neighbourhood;

- having an adequate income;

- maintaining a sense of independence and control over one's life.

Respondents often commented on the multi-faceted nature of QoL, and the interdependency of its components. For example, retaining one's independence and social participation were often described as being dependent on retaining good health and an adequate financial situation, as well as access to transport. These can also be influenced by social and community resources, as well as one's psychological characteristics. Overall, this research showed that most respondents enjoyed the flexibility of retirement, and freedom from the time constraints of paid work, but these could only be really enjoyed if relatively good health was maintained, if people had enough money and lived in areas which facilitated social relationships, neighbourliness, activity and mobility. Greater recognition is needed in definitions of QoL, and its measurement, that influencing variables include people's own characteristics and circumstances, their individual interpretations and priorities, and the dynamic interplay between people and their surrounding social structures in a changing society. Thus, broad, rather than single-model (see Chapter 1) theoretical approaches are needed in order to understand the experience of ageing, and QoL in older age.

The positive circumstances and attitudes of older people, and the identification of a common core of values for QoL, however, should not deflect attention from the negative circumstances and attitudes of sizeable minorities, and society's responsibility towards them, or obscure the diversity of older people. While there was considerable consensus on the main constituents of what gave life quality, different priorities emerged depending on whether people were questioned about the good or bad areas of life quality, priorities and suggestions for improvements. For example, while having good social relationships was the most commonly mentioned constituent that gave people's lives quality, poor health, living in poor housing and neighbourhoods and not having enough money were the most often mentioned things that took quality away. And both health and money were the most often mentioned as the most important areas of quality of life overall. Having health, followed by having enough money, were the most often mentioned areas when people were asked about what single thing would improve the quality of their own lives. However, finance, *followed* by health, was most often mentioned as the single thing that would improve the lives of other people their age. The descriptive analyses also indicated, in particular, that, not only were incomes often very low, for many there was also a feeling of not being safe walking alone outdoors at night and, although ratings of the facilities in neighbourhoods were generally positive, poorer ratings were given overall to local social and leisure facilities, facilities for people aged 65+, transport and closeness to shops. These are essential elements of social capital which enable social participation and involvement in communities (see Chapter 7).There were also differences in the QoL themes mentioned by men and women, and by people in younger and older age groups. For example, it was shown in Chapter 3 that women were more likely than men to mention home and neighbourhood, social relationships and social activities as giving their life quality, whereas men were more likely to mention finances and independence, perhaps reflecting traditional gender role divisions. People aged 75+ were more likely than younger respondents to mention health, home and neighbourhood as giving life quality.

Further comment about the contribution of psychological outlook is needed. Relative deprivation theory holds that happiness, well-being and QoL partly depend on what people have relative to a norm, which is affected by what others have. If people make downward social comparisons of themselves and their circumstances with others who are worse off than them, they are likely to be happier and more satisfied with their situation than people who make upward comparisons with people who are better off. The data reported in Chapters 3 and 6 supported the need to avoid making unrealistic upward comparisons, as this can only lead to dissatisfaction and worse perceived QoL. Those who made downward social comparisons with those who were worse off had better psychological health (GHQ scores). However, the data also showed that those on the lowest incomes were most likely to make upward comparisons. Inevitably, those on the lowest incomes may find downward comparisons more difficult, and downward comparisons may be an unrealistic suggestion for some groups. But despite their relatively low incomes, only a minority of respondents felt that they were worse off than they had expected to be, and many had optimistic outlooks on life. This is likely to partly reflect low expectations and their standards for making social comparisons. As the subject for comparison was often a hypothetical group ('i.e. people my own age'), low expectations of older age contributed to their perceptions. While positive psychology might encourage people to make downward social comparisons for their enhanced well-being, they should not be encouraged to have unrealistically low expectations which can only disadvantage their experiences and achievements throughout life. Higher expectations would be productive if they led to a more demanding public. For example, this could be to the benefit of older people if it resulted in less age discrimination in society (e.g. in access to appropriate health services) (Bowling 1999, 2002; Bowling *et al.* 2001; Bond *et al.* 2003).

Traditional sociological theory holds that well-being depends on one's socio-economic position in society. It has been argued that, for those in disadvantaged social positions, including those in retirement and older age groups, this status adds to their sense of powerlessness and loss of control (Phillipson 1987; Fennell *et al.* 1988). Less than half of the respondents in the QoL survey felt they had a lot of control over their lives, although just under two-thirds scored middle to high for self-efficacy overall. As pointed out above, self-efficacy was found to be influenced by socioeconomic position. People with the highest socioeconomic status (with the highest level of education, the highest incomes, in the highest social classes, and those who are home owners) were advantaged by being more likely to have the highest self-efficacy. Similarly, the direction of social comparisons was affected by level of income. Thus, there are likely to be socioeconomic barriers to the promotion of psychological resources in individuals. There is evidence from other studies that one's outlook is associated with the place occupied in the status hierarchy (Marmot 2004). This is an issue that has been neglected by positive psychologists.

Significance of the findings for QoL research

The results of the research presented here show that it is important to develop a model of QoL for use in both descriptive and evaluative research (e.g. in health and social policy) which reflects the views of the population concerned, and encompasses individuals' values. QoL instruments should focus on far more than the traditional areas of life satisfaction, or health and physical functioning, in order to gain a better understanding of the quality of later life. QoL, from the perspective of older people, is more multi-dimensional and dynamic than most 'expert' views, which are often based on a limited number of domains. Moreover, within each QoL theme mentioned by older people, there were many different reasons given about why that area was important to them (see sub-themes in Annex I, Chapter 3) (see also Bowling *et al.* 2003; Bowling and Gabriel 2004). This diversity of views was also reported by Stenner *et al.* (2003), who explored individuals' different constructions of questions from their World Health Organization Quality of Life (WHOQoL) questionnaire. They concluded that this variation in interpretation needs to be considered when developing subjective scales of QoL and in their testing for reliability. Much greater recognition of the different values people place on different components of QoL is needed in research. As Walker (2005) argued, the dominant 'expert' approach to assessing QoL has wrongly tended to homogenize older people, and to perceive old age as detached from other phases of life (resulting in old age being regarded as a 'problem').

While the call for a broader model of QoL is not new (Cella and Tulsky 1990), many of the themes identified in this study have still been omitted in recently developed models and measures (WHOQOL Group 1993; Skevington 1999; Skevington *et al.* 1999). In particular, as indicated earlier, the multi-faceted nature of independence autonomy and control, and their enabling factors, particularly in older age, are generally neglected in the wider measurement literature. Commonly used measures of the ability to perform activities of daily living, instrumental activities and mobility only cover physical ability and independence in functioning. Likewise, many of the other sub-themes reported in this study have received little attention in the QoL conceptual and measurement literature – for example, the enjoyment of one's home, the importance of the wider social capital, access to public transport, being able to drive and maintain a car for enabling continued independence, social participation and enjoyment of life in older age. And, again, influencing variables include a dynamic interplay between people's individual characteristics and their surrounding social structures in a changing society (White-Riley and Riley 1999). This calls for longitudinal and repeated cross-sectional research, with designs that can take life changes, response shift (Sprangers and Schwartz 1999), and the effects of ageing into account, as well as individual values, perceptions, characteristics and circumstances. The latter is essential in order to address the issue of whether attempting to engineer gains in subjective QoL is a realistic policy goal, in view of the potential influence of personality on perceived well-being (Lykken and Tellegen 1996).

While people apply their individual meanings to situations, they are, of course, also influenced by their personal history, experiences, education and the structure of the society they live in. The current generation of people aged over 50 are the next generation of older people and their demands and aspirations may be quite different. They include the post Second World War baby boomers who will have a higher level of education and higher incomes and most of whom will have occupational pensions with accompanying increased purchasing power. Their expectations are likely to be different from the current generation of older people in Britain who experienced the depression in the 1930s and a world war. Many of this age group left school at 14, with no further qualifications and are reliant on a state pension and benefits (Nelson *et al.* 2001). Longitudinal research is needed to assess both cohort effects and the effects of changing values on QoL. Further research is needed on the dynamics of QoL, the interdependency of domains, the distinction between indicator and causal variables (Fayers and Hand 2002) and potential mediating variables (Zizzi *et al.* 1998). An appreciation of these issues would lead to more appropriate measurement scales. This is the next step that is needed in QoL research.

How QoL in older age can be improved

The results from each methodological approach to investigating QoL gave valuable indicators about how QoL might generally be improved in older age for both men and women. Respondents emphasized the importance to their QoL of having good health, independence, social relationships and participation, maintaining a positive outlook, having enough money, of living in a neighbourly area. Also important were having access to good local facilities, including shops, transport and places to meet other people and socialize, opportunities for participation in voluntary work, good local health and council services, and having pleasant, safe surroundings. The results also showed that most people placed a high value on their health. They understood that health is a key component of a good QoL, and that it acts as the 'foundation' of other aspects of life. Health has been called a 'special good' (Berlin 1969), as inequalities in health in older age lead to inequalities in functioning, social participation, activity and independence. This strengthens the case for ensuring equity of access to health services by age (Bowling *et al.* 2002b). And given that socioeconomic factors influence health, as well as psychological resources, albeit over a lifetime, society also has a collective responsibility to ensure that retirement pensions are adequate.

Hartman-Stein and Potkanowicz (2003) reviewed the literature on the predictors of successful ageing and stated that there is evidence that behaviour at age 50 is likely to affect how people feel at age 80. In particular, behaviours that prevent disease-related disability, cognitive impairment and late life depression included regular physical exercise, engaging in cognitively stimulating activities, maintaining and optimistic mental outlook and finding meaning in life. While most people in the QoL survey described themselves as optimistic, and there was evidence of much social activity, only about a fifth were engaged in exercises involving physical exertion, such as physical sports or keeping fit. More reported less demanding physical activities: about two-thirds reported going for walks, and almost six in ten reported gardening as one of their activities. National statistics also show that walking is the most popular physical activity among people aged 65+ (Walker *et al.* 2001). Fewer respondents improved their minds by formally attending educational classes, or through hobbies which exercised their minds (e.g. crosswords, bingo). These results suggest that there is scope for providing more focused activities, aimed at maintaining physical strength and aerobic capacity, for the current generation of people aged 65 and over. Local authorities in the UK could examine initiatives elsewhere in Europe aimed at enabling older people to continue to participate socially in society. For example, in Jyväskylä, Finland, local authorities became concerned about older people staying indoors during the winter, when it was dark and pavements were slippery. They therefore negotiated with local bus companies to organize bus travel from 17 regions, stopping at day centres, residential care homes and swimming pools. The bus fares were paid for by the swimming pools and older people participated mainly in aqua-aerobics. There are lessons here, given the evidence from this study and other surveys showing that large numbers of older people in Britain do not venture out at night due to concerns about their safety, and find public transport inadequate or too expensive. Such self-imposed curfews are socially created, and result in limitations to people's independence, social participation and activities, social networks and contacts, and ultimately their well-being and QoL.

Most respondents already had full lives in other areas. They often commented on coping with older age by keeping busy, and often appeared to fill their lives with activity. Being socially active was seen by people as not only preventing loneliness, but as a main part of QoL. Almost a fifth to a quarter of respondents were also engaged in helping others, through babysitting, looking after grandchildren, looking after someone who is ill or frail, and voluntary work. These figures are similar to those from large US surveys (e.g. Offer 1997), but higher than those reported by Marmot *et al.* (2003) from the 2002 English Longitudinal Survey of Ageing, but may reflect differences in question wording. And, of course, most older people are women, who continue to perform conventional, essential domestic tasks for themselves and others (e.g. for their spouses) (see Thane 2000). Far from being burdens, older people are often valuable and reciprocal contributors to their families and society.

People of all ages, of course, could also be encouraged to develop and maintain social relationships and activities throughout their lives, given their importance to QoL, and given that these decline in number, rather than accumulate, in older age. But they also need to be facilitated in this by the provision of local facilities which promote a sense of community, as well as encouraging social contacts, roles and activities. Some circumstances are not within the power of all individuals to influence – for example, the level of pensions and other retirement income, available and accessible transport or the quality and perceived safety of one's home and neighbourhood. These are areas for further policy consideration.

Can people build up their psychological resources? As one grows older, the need to be strong increases in the face of adversity and loss. It was pointed out in Chapters 1 and 6 that the employment of psychological resources is important for success when facing the dynamic between life's challenges and depleting reserves. The use of self-enhancing social comparisons (e.g. when in poor health) has been suggested as one strategy for maintaining self-esteem and well-being (Ryff 1999). Another is the use of 'selective optimization with compensation' (Baltes and Baltes 1990b). For example, when selected activities have to be discarded (e.g. due to ill-health or bereavement) strategies need to be activated in order to find new ones and to maximize the chances of maintaining reserves. There is some supportive evidence that these strategies are associated with higher levels of life satisfaction and QoL, (Freund and Baltes 1998).

Older people interviewed for this survey demonstrated considerable coping skills when faced with declining health, lower income and the loss of spouses, relatives and friends through death. People spoke of their own personalities, attitudes and philosophies on life as affecting their QoL, as these influenced their interpretation of their current circumstances and past life events. Their coping strategies were said to include acceptance of life, making downward social comparisons, 'feeling lucky' and having an optimistic outlook. Some spoke of actively 'making their own QoL' by 'keeping busy' and seeking out social and leisure activities which gave them satisfaction, and of finding new activities when they were no longer able to continue with usual interests due to ill-health. Social comparisons and expectations, and level of optimism, were among the main independent predictors of perceived QoL in the regression model, although self-efficacy (self-mastery) did not retain significance in the final model.

There is an increasing popular literature on the self-promotion of psychological well-being. Positive affect (e.g. feeling hopeful about the future, being self-confident, having enjoyment of life – see Ostir *et al.* 2004) is widely recognized as having protective benefits against poor health and physical functioning, including reduction of risk of medical events such as stroke and myocardial infarction (Segerstrom *et al.* 1998; Ostir *et al.* 2000, 2001a, 2001b).

In this study, positive outlook was associated with better psychological health and with good QoL. Positive psychologists, reminiscent of positive-thinking movements, believe that optimism can be learned, and that having a happy outlook can be cultivated. Avoidance of focusing on negative thoughts is argued to be insufficient alone to promote a positive mood – positive thoughts are also needed. Seligman (2004) argued that one has to identify and use one's signature strengths and traits (e.g. kindness, originality, humour, optimism, generosity) to be happy, and that once people are aware of these they find life more gratifying and develop natural buffers against stress and life events. It should be remembered, however, that getting people to 'cheer up' is not easily achieved in real life. Moreover, it has been postulated that there is a dispositional effect on perceived QoL. As pointed out in Chapter 1, Lykken and Tellegen (1996) argued, on the basis of their twin studies, that up to around half of the variance in well-being was associated with genetic variation rather than social circumstances, which potentially limits suggestions for self-development. However, this remains an unresolved issue.

The QoL themes which emerged from this research are all areas relevant to health and social policy, and where targets for action and audit could be set. This research illustrated the interdependency of different areas of life. Public policy departments tend to regard their own areas in isolation of others, while the promotion of well-being requires that interdependencies and knock-on effects are understood and taken into account. Age Concern England's (2003) policy report on the findings of this survey emphasized the need for local and central government to undertake several approaches. These included the need to assess the impact on the QoL of older people of current government policies and programmes on pensions, health services and neighbourhood renewal and action; to develop the capacity of older people themselves and encourage their involvement in community consultation processes; to support the voluntary sector in its promotion of social inclusion and social relationships among this group; and to encourage the social inclusion of older people by tackling barriers to participation which include age discrimination as well as problems of taxation and insurance.

Finally, the next generations of older and retired people, including those born between 1945 and 1965, are likely to be more radical than the current generation, and become major campaigning groups. The 17 million people in Britain who grew up with peace movements, the women's liberation movement, anti-racism, environmentalism and in the vanguard of the sexual revolution are approaching retirement. They have been the first generation to grow up in a strong consumer-oriented society and have been led to expect the satisfaction of their needs. In fact, because of their vast numbers, the next generation of older people is likely to be more economically and politically powerful than the current one. They are anticipated to be more demanding, active, liberal in attitude and have higher expectations of life (Huber and Skidmore 2003; Harkin and Huber 2004). On the basis of consumer research in Britain and the USA, and focus group interviews in England, Harkin and Huber (2004) reported that the baby boomers were refusing to age in a stereo-typical manner, and saw retirement as a time for adventurous travel. Scales and Scase (2000) also reported that people currently aged in their 50s have active and hedonistic views of their retirement. This generation is particularly likely to promote active ageing more vigorously than any other preceding it. While it has been argued that governments ignore them at their peril, it is, as yet, unknown whether this particular generation will use their voting power to promote their own interests or push for wider social change (Huber and Skidmore 2003).

Glossary

active ageing continuing physical, psychological, social health, participation, independence, autonomy, control for the enhancement of quality of life.

activities of daily living (ADL) personal care tasks such as eating/drinking, washing self, using the toilet, rising from a chair, getting in/out of bed, moving around indoors, dressing, walking outdoors.

activity, or role, theory maintenance of social roles and activities that are meaningful to people and enhance feelings of well-being in older age.

age identity how old people actually feel in relation to their actual age (see also subjective age).

age stratification theory there is an age structure to roles, and normative age criteria for certain activities, thus with age a cohort moves to a different set of roles as a younger generation takes its place.

autonomy being free to make decisions for oneself and implement these.

biological ageing the progressive constriction of each organ's capacity to maintain homoeostasis when challenged, leading to reduced physiological adaptability, increased susceptibility and vulnerability to disease and eventually death.

carer a person who supports and has most contact with a dependent older person and is not paid for their work.

chronological age the use of specific birth anniversaries to define old age; this is increasingly regarded as inadequate for this purpose.

confidant someone close with whom private matters can be confided, or who offers emotional support and comfort.

compression of morbidity hypothesis morbidity in old age will be compressed into a shorter time span, perhaps due to healthier lifestyles or medical advances.

continuity theory individuals make adaptations to enable them to feel the continuity between the past and present, which preserves psychological well-being.

control being able to manage (control) one's life, and its demands, while also being aware that there are areas of life outside one's control.

dependency the extent to which a person needs help from others to maintain a normal life.

disability inability to perform tasks and functions in a normal manner (see activities of daily living and instrumental activities of daily living).

disability-free life expectancy mortality and morbidity data for a population are aggregated into a single index, representing the average number of years that a person of a given age may expect to live free of disability.

disengagement theory gradual withdrawal from social interactions and activities is an inevitable accompaniment of older age; this protects the individual against the trauma of dying and minimizes disruption to society when death takes place.

effect size a numerical index of the magnitude of an observed association.

fourth age the period of increasing frailty before death.

handicap the social disadvantage or loss of role associated with disease.

health-related quality of life (HRQoL) an amorphous concept and a wide range of pertinent domains have been identified in the literature, including the perceived impact of health on optimum levels of physical, psychological and social well-being and functioning, level of independence, and satisfaction with these levels.

health status perceived physical, psychological and social health.

healthy survivor effect bias due the operation of some selective survival of the fittest into old age.

impairment, disability and handicap the ways in which chronic diseases have an impact on the individual (World Health Organization 1980); since revised more positively to impairments, activities and participation (World Health Organization 1998).

independence acting for oneself, as in physical ability, the ability to organize one's day-to-day life and so on.

instrumental activities of daily living (IADL) household, rather than personal, management activities: preparing meals, bed-making, laundry/ironing, managing money, using the telephone, shopping and heavy housework.

life expectancy the average (median) number of years that a person can expect to live, usually based on contemporary death rates which may be higher than those experienced by future cohorts, so tends to underestimate life expectancy.

modernization theory with the emergence of new technology, which undermined the status of older people through the emphasis on education, rather than older adults passing on knowledge and skills, they lost their place of prestige and power within the social system.

old age usually defined arbitrarily in relation to a specific birth anniversary, often coinciding with an official age of retirement (see chronological age).

positive ageing see successful ageing.

quality of life (QoL) a multi-level and amorphous concept, broadly defined as encompassing the individual's perceptions of, and satisfaction with, physical health, psychological well-being, independence, social relationships, social and material circumstances and the natural and built environments; ultimately dependent on the perceptions of the individual.

response shift internal standards and values change between different points in time (e.g. baseline and follow-up surveys) affecting perceptions of life circumstances (e.g. QoL).

retirement age inability or choice not to remain in paid employment associated with reaching a certain age (varies between 50 and 70 years).

self-efficacy or self-mastery the ability to maintain some control over life, and a changing view of life, in a way that preserves a sense of control when faced with the changes and limitations that can accompany ageing.

self-mastery see self-efficacy.

social capital the collective value of formal and informal social networks, and the enabling facilities of community resources.

social competence the employment of compensatory strategies when facing the dynamic between challenges and depleting reserves.

social exchange theory the cost-benefit ratio between the individual and society falls out of balance in older age, thus the costs of interacting with older people outweigh the benefits.

social handicap barriers to participation and independent functioning imposed by society.

social network the set of links between identified groups of people.

social support the interactive process through which emotional and instrumental aid, information and guidance is received from one's social network.

structured dependency old age is structured by the dominant economic and political forces.

subjective age how old people actually feel in relation to their actual age (see age identity).

successful ageing definitions range from reaching one's potential, achieving physical, psychological and social well-being, including life satisfaction, the ability to adapt one's values to meet the challenges of later life, having the physiological and psychological abilities of younger people and engaging with life, cognitive efficiency, social competence and skills, self-mastery, adaptation, control and maintenance of productivity and achievement.

third age a continuation of life in which retirement, in theory, enables citizens to live at leisure and realize their ambitions (not available for people on low incomes or in poor health).

triangulation the use of more than one research method (usually three or more) within a study.

utilitarianism production of the greatest possible total happiness, good or 'utility' of the greatest number of people.

See also Bowling and Ebrahim (2001).

References

Abbey, A. and Andrews, F.M. (1985) Modelling the psychological determinants of life quality, *Social Indicators Research*, 16: 1–34.

Abbey, A. and Andrews, F.M. (1986) Modelling the psychological determinants of life quality, in F.M. Andrews (ed.) *Research on the Quality of Life*. Ann Arbor, MI: Survey Research Center, Institute for Social Research, University of Michigan.

Abeles, R.P. (1991) Personal autonomy for residents in long-term care – concepts and issues of measurement, in J.E. Birren, J.E. Lubben, J.C. Rowe and D.E. Deutchman (eds) *The Concept and Measurement of Quality of Life in the Frail Elderly*. San Diego, CA: Academic Press.

Adamson, J., Hunt, K. and Ebrahim, S. (2003) Socioeconomic position, occupational exposures, and gender: the relation with locomotor disability in early old age, *Journal of Epidemiology and Community Health*, 57: 453–5.

Affleck, G. (1987) Downward comparison and coping with serious medical problems, *American Journal of Orthopsychiatry*, 57: 570–8.

Age Concern England (1992) *Dependence: The Ultimate Fear*. London: Age Concern England.

Age Concern England (2003) *Adding Quality to Quantity: Older People's Views on Quality of Life and its Enhancement*, compiled by A. Bowling and C. Kennelly. London: Age Concern England.

Age Concern England (2004) *LifeForce Programme*. London: Age Concern Research Services.

Albrecht, G.L. and Devlieger, P.J. (1999) The disability paradox: high quality of life against all odds, *Social Science and Medicine*, 48: 977–88.

Anand, S. (2002) The concern for equity in health, *Journal of Epidemiology and Community Health*, 56: 485–7.

Andrews, F.M. (1973) *List of Social Concerns Common to Most OECD Countries*. Paris: OECD.

Andrews, F.M. (1974) Social indicators of perceived life quality, *Social Indicators Research*, 1: 279–99.

Andrews, F.M. (ed.) (1986) *Research on the Quality of Life*. University of Michigan: Institute for Social Research.

Andrews, F.M. and Crandall, R. (1976) The validity of measures of self-reported well-being, *Social Indicators Research*, 3: 1–19.

Andrews, F.M. and McKennel, A.C. (1980) Measures of self-reported well-being: their affective, cognitive and other components, *Social Indicators Research*, 18: 127–55.

Andrews, F.M. and Withey, S.B. (1976a) *Social Indicators of Well-being: American's Perceptions of Life Quality*. New York: Plenum Press.

Andrews, F.M. and Withey, S.B. (1976b) Developing measures of perceived life quality: results from several national surveys, *Social Indicators Research*, 1: 1–26.

Andrews, G., Clark, M. and Luszcz, M. (2002) Successful aging in the Australian Longitudinal Study of Aging: applying the MacArthur model cross-nationally, *Journal of Social Issues*, 58: 749–65.

Antonovsky, A. (1987) *Unravelling the Mystery of Health: How People Manage Stress and Stay Well*. San Francisco: Jossey-Bass.

Antonucci, T. and Jackson, J. (1989) Successful ageing and life course reciprocity, in A.M. Warnes (ed.) *Human Ageing and Later Life*. London: Edward Arnold.

Argyle, M. (1996) Subjective well-being, in A. Offer (ed.) *In Pursuit of the Quality of Life*. Oxford: Oxford University Press.

Argyle, M., Martin, M. and Crossland, J. (1989) Happiness as a function of personality and social encounters, in J.P. Forgas and J.M. Innes (eds) *Recent Advances in Social Psychology: An International Perspective*. North Holland: Elsevier Science.

Arnold, S. (1991) Measurement of quality of life in the frail elderly, in J.E. Birren, J.E. Lubben and J.C. Rowe (eds) *The Concept and Measurement of Quality of Life in the Frail Elderly*. San Diego, CA: Academic Press.

Atchley, R. (1989) A continuity theory of normal aging, *The Gerontologist*, 29: 183–90.

Atchley, R. (1999) *Continuity and Adaptation in Aging: Creating Positive Experiences*. Baltimore, MD: Johns Hopkins University Press.

Attwood, C., Singh, G., Prime, D. *et al.* (2003) *2001 Citizenship Survey: People, Families and Communities*, Home Office Research Study 270. London: Home Office.

Audit Commission (2002) *Quality of Life: Using Quality of Life Indicators*. London: Audit Commission.

Avlund, K., Holstein, B.E., Damsgaard, M.T. *et al.* (2003) Social position and health in old age: the relevance of different indicators of social position, *Scandanavian Journal of Public Health*, 31: 126–36.

Ayis, S., Gooberman-Hill, R. and Ebrahim, S. (2003) Long-standing and limiting long-standing illness in older people: associations with chronic diseases, psychosocial and environmental factors, *Age and Ageing*, 32: 265–72.

Baltes, M.M., Mayer, M., Borchelt, M. *et al.* (1996) Everyday competence in old and very old age: an interdisciplinary perspective, *Ageing and Society*, 13: 657–80.

Baltes, P.B. and Baltes, M.M. (eds) (1990a) *Successful Aging: Perspectives from the Behavioral Sciences*. New York: Cambridge University Press.

Baltes, P.B. and Baltes, M.M. (1990b) Psychological perspectives on successful aging: the model of selective optimisation with compensation, in P.B. Baltes and M.M. Baltes (eds) *Successful Aging: Perspectives from the Behavioral Sciences*. New York: Cambridge University Press.

Baltes, P.B. and Smith, J. (2003) New frontiers in the future of ageing: from successful ageing of young old to the dilemmas of the fourth age, *Gerontology*, 49: 123–35.

Bandura, A. (1977) Self-efficacy: toward a unifying theory of behavioral change, *Psychological Review*, 84: 191–215.

Banister, D. and Bowling, A. (2004) Quality of life and the elderly: the transport dimension, *Transport Policy*, 11: 105–15.

Barak, B. and Schiffman, L. (1981) Cognitive age: a nonchronological age variable, in K. Monroe (ed.) *Advances in Consumer Research*. Ann Arbor, MI: Association for Consumer Research.

Barry, M.M. (1997) Well-being and life satisfaction as components of quality of life in mental disorders, in H. Katschnig, H. Freeman and N. Sartorius (eds) *Quality of Life in Mental Disorders*. Chichester: Wiley.

Bauer, R.A. (1966) *Social Indicators*. Cambridge, MA: MIT Press.

Beaumont, J.G. and Kenealy, P.M. (2004) Quality of life perceptions and social comparisons in healthy old age, *Ageing and Society*, 24: 755–69.

Bearon, L.B. (1996) Successful aging: what does the 'good life' look like? *The Forum for Family and Consumer Issues, North Carolina State University*, 1: 1–6.

Beck, A.M. and Meyers, N.M. (1996) Health enhancement and companion animal ownership, *Annual Review of Public Health*, 17: 247–57.

Beckie, T.M. and Hayduk, L.A. (1997) Measuring quality of life, *Social Indicators Research*, 42: 21–39.

Bentham, J. (1834) *Deonotology*. Oxford: Clarendon Press.

Berkman, C. and Gurland, B.J. (1998) The relationship among income, other socioeconomic indicators, and functional level in older persons, *Journal of Aging and Health*, 10: 81–98.

Berkman, L.F. and Breslow, L. (1983) *Health and Ways of Living: The Alameida County Study*. New York: Oxford University Press.

Berkman, L.F. and Glass, T. (2000) Social integration, social networks, social support and health, in L.F. Berkman and I. Kawachi (eds) *Social Epidemiology*. Oxford: Oxford University Press.

Berkman, L.F. and Syme, S.L. (1979) Social networks, host resistance and mortality: a nine-year follow-up of Alameda County residents, *American Journal of Epidemiology*, 109: 186–204.

Berkman, L.F., Leo-Summers, L. and Horowitz, R.I. (1992) Emotional support and survival after myocardial infarction: a prospective, population-based study of the elderly, *Annals of Internal Medicine*, 117: 1003–9.

Berlin, I. (1969) *Four Essays on Liberty*. Oxford: Oxford University Press.

Bierman, B.S., Bubolz, T.A. and Elliott, A. (1999) How well does a single question about health predict the financial health of Medicare managed care plans? *Effective Clinical Practice*, 2: 56–62.

Bigelow, D.A., Brodsky, G., Steward, L. and Olson, M.M. (1982) The concept and measurement of quality of life as a dependent variable in evaluation of mental health services, in G.J. Stahler and W.R. Tash (eds) *Innovative Approaches to Mental Health Evaluation*. New York: Academic Press.

Bigelow, D.A., McFarlane, B.H. and Olson, M.M. (1991) Quality of life of community mental health programme clients: validating a measure, *Community Mental Health Journal*, 27: 43–55.

Blacksher, E. (2002) On being poor and feeling poor: low socioeconomic status and the moral self, *Theory Medical Bioethics*, 23: 455–70.

Blaikie, A. (1999) *Ageing and Popular Culture*. Cambridge: Cambridge University Press.

Blalock, S.J., De Vellis, B.M. and De Vellis, R.F. (1989) Social comparison among individuals with rheumatoid arthritis, *Journal of Applied Social Psychology*, 19: 665–80.

Blalock, S.J., De Vellis, B.M. and De Vellis, R.F. (1990) Adjustment to rheumatoid arthritis: the role of social comparison processes, *Health Education Research*, 5: 361–70.

Blanchflower, D.G. and Oswald, A.J. (2001) *Well-being Over Time in Britain and the USA*. Warwick: University of Warwick, research paper no. 616, Department of Economics.

Blane, D., Wiggins, R., Higgs, P. and Hyde, M. (2002) *Inequalities in Quality of Life in Early Old Age*, GO Findings no. 9. Sheffield: Growing Older Programme.

Blane, D., Higgs, P., Hyde, M. and Wiggins, R.D. (2004) Life course influences on quality of life in early old age, *Social Science and Medicine*, 58: 2171–9.

Blau, P.M. (1964) *Exchange and Power in Social Life*. New York: Wiley.

Blau, Z.S. (1973) *Old Age in a Changing Society*. New York: Watts.

Blazer, D.G. (1982) Social support and mortality in an elderly community population, *American Journal of Epidemiology*, 115: 684–94.

Blazer, D. (2002) Self-efficacy and depression in late life: a primary prevention proposal, *Ageing and Mental Health*, 6: 315–24.

Boaz, A., Hayden, C. and Bernard, M. (1999) *Attitudes and Aspirations of Older People: A Review of the Literature*, research report no. 1. London: Department of Social Security.

Boelhouwer, J. (2002) Quality of life and living conditions in the Netherlands, *Social Indicators Research*, 58: 113–38.

Bond, J. and Carstairs, V. (1982) *Services for the Elderly: A Survey of the Characteristics and Needs of a Population of 5,000,000 Old People*, Scottish Home and Health Studies no. 42. Edinburgh: Scottish Home and Health Department.

Bond, J. and Corner, L. (2004) *Quality of Life and Older People*. Maidenhead: Open University Press.

Bond, M., Bowling, A., McKee, D. *et al.* (2003) Is age a predictor of access to cardiac services? *Journal of Health Services Research and Policy*, 8: 40–7.

Boots Company (2002) *Well-being Customer Survey*. Nottingham: Boots Company.

Bowling, A. (1987) Mortality after bereavement: a review of the literature on survival periods and factors affecting survival, *Social Science and Medicine*, 24: 117–24.

Bowling, A. (1988) Who dies after widow(er)hood? A discriminant analysis, *Omega, Journal of Death and Dying*, 19: 135–53.

Bowling, A. (1990) The prevalence of psychiatric morbidity among people aged 85 and over living at home, *Social Psychiatry and Psychiatric Epidemiology*, 25: 132–40.

Bowling, A. (1991) Social support and social networks: their relationship to the successful and unsuccessful survival of elderly people in the community. An analysis of concepts and a review of the evidence, *Family Practice*, 8: 68–83.

Bowling, A. (1993) The concepts of successful and positive ageing, *Family Practice*, 10: 449–53.

Bowling, A. (1994) Social networks and social support among older people and implications for emotional well-being and psychiatric morbidity, *International Review of Psychiatry*, 9: 447–59.

Bowling, A. (1995a) What things are important in people's lives? *Social Science and Medicine*, 41: 1447–62.

Bowling, A. (1995b) The most important things in life: comparisons between older and younger population age groups by gender, *International Journal of Health Sciences*, 6: 169–75.

Bowling, A. (1996) The effects of illness on quality of life, *Journal of Epidemiology and Community Health*, 50: 149–55.

Bowling, A. (1999) Ageism in cardiology, *British Medical Journal*, 319: 1353–5.

Bowling, A. (2001) *Measuring Disease: A Review of Disease Specific Measurement Scales*, 2nd edn. Buckingham: Open University Press.

Bowling, A. (2002) An 'inverse satisfaction' law? Why don't older patients criticise health services? Speaker's corner, *Journal of Epidemiology and Community Health*, 56: 482.

Bowling, A. (2004a) *Measuring Health: A Review of Quality of Life Measurement Scales*, 3rd edn. Maidenhead: Open University Press.

Bowling, A. (2004b) Socio-economic differentials in mortality among older people, *Journal of Epidemiology and Community Health*, 58: 438–40.

Bowling, A. (2005) Techniques of questionnaire design, in A. Bowling and S. Ebrahim (eds) *Handbook of Health Research Methods: Investigation, Measurement and Analysis*. Maidenhead: Open University Press.

Bowling, A. and Browne, P. (1991) Social networks, health and emotional well-being among the oldest old living in London, *Journal of Gerontology*, 46: S20–32.

Bowling, A. and Cartwright, A. (1982) *Life After a Death: A Study of the Elderly Widowed*. London: Tavistock.

Bowling, A. and Charlton, J. (1987) Mortality after bereavement: a logistic regression analysis, *Journal of the Royal College of General Practitioners*, 37: 551–4.

Bowling, A. and Ebrahim, S. (2001) Glossaries in public health: older people, *Journal of Epidemiology and Community Health*, 55: 223–6.

Bowling, M. and Farquhar, M. (1991) Associations with social networks, social support, health status and psychiatric morbidity in three samples of elderly people, *Social Psychiatry and Psychiatric Epidemiology*, 26: 115–26.

Bowling, A. and Gabriel, Z. (2004) An integrational model of quality of life in older age: a comparison of analytic and lay models of quality of life, *Social Indicators Research*, 69: 1–36.

Bowling, A. and Grundy, E. (1998) Longitudinal studies of social networks and mortality in later life, *Reviews in Clinical Gerontology*, 8: 353–61.

Bowling, A. and Windsor, J. (1995) Death after widow(er)hood: an analysis of mortality rates up to 13 years after bereavement, *Omega Journal of Death and Dying*, 31: 35–49.

Bowling, A. and Windsor, J. (2001) Towards the good life: a population survey of dimensions of quality of life, *Journal of Happiness Studies*, 2: 55–81.

Bowling, A., Edelmann, R.J., Leaver, J. and Hoeckel, T. (1989) Loneliness, mobility, well-being and social support in a sample of over 85 year olds, *Journal of Personality and Individual Differences*, 10: 1189–92.

Bowling, A., Farquhar, M. and Browne, P. (1991) Life satisfaction and associations with social network and support variables in three samples of elderly people, *International Journal of Geriatric Psychiatry*, 6: 549–66.

Bowling, A., Farquhar, M. and Grundy, E. (1994) Changes in the ability to get outdoors among a community sample of people aged 85+ in 1987: results from a follow-up study in 1990, *International Journal of Health Sciences*, 5: 13–23.

Bowling, A., Farquhar, M. and Grundy, E. (1995a) Changes in network composition among older people living in inner London and Essex, *Journal of Health and Place*, 1: 149–66.

Bowling, A., Farquhar, M. and Grundy, E. (1995b) Changes in network composition among the very old living in inner London, *Journal of Cross-Cultural Gerontology*, 10: 331–47.

Bowling, A., Farquhar, M. and Grundy, E. (1996) Associations with changes in life satisfaction among three samples of elderly people living at home, *International Journal of Geriatric Psychiatry*, 11: 1077–87.

Bowling, A., Farquhar, M., Grundy, E. and Formby, J. (1999) Changes in life satisfaction over a two and a half year period among very elderly people living in London, *Social Science and Medicine*, 36: 641–55.

Bowling, A., Bond, M., McKee, D. *et al.* (2001) Equity in access to exercise tolerance testing, coronary angiography, and coronary artery bypass grafting by age, sex and clinical indications, *Heart*, 85: 680–6.

Bowling, A., Banister, D., Sutton, S. *et al.* (2002a) A multidimensional model of QoL in older age, *Ageing and Mental Health*, 6: 355–71.

Bowling, A., Mariotto, A. and Evans, O. (2002b) Are older people willing to give up their place in the queue for cardiac surgery to a younger person? *Age and Ageing*, 31: 187–92.

Bowling, A., Gabriel, Z., Dykes, J. et al. (2003) Let's ask them: a national survey of definitions of quality of life and its enhancement among people aged 65 and over, *International Journal of Aging and Human Development*, 56: 269–306.

Bowling A., Seetai, S., Ebrahim, S., Gabriel, Z. and Solanki, P. (2005) Attributes of age-identity, *Ageing and Society*, 25: 479–500.

Bradburn, N.M. (1969) *The Structure of Psychological Well-being*. Chicago: Aldine Press.

Bradburn, N.M. and Caplowitz, D. (1965) *Reports on Happiness*. Chicago: Aldine Press.

Brandstadter, J. and Greve, W. (1994) The aging self: stabilizing the protective process, *Developmental Review*, 14: 52–80.

Brandstadler, J. and Renner, G. (1990) Tenacious goal pursuit and flexible goal adjustment: explication and age-related analysis of assimilative and accommodative strategies of coping, *Psychology and Aging*, 5: 58–67.

Breeze, E., Grundy, C., Fletcher, A. et al. (2001) *Inequalities in Quality of Life Among People Aged 75 Years and Over in Great Britain*. Sheffield: ESRC Growing Older Programme, Research Findings 1.

Breeze, E., Jones, D.A., Wilkinson, P. et al. (2004) Association with quality of life in old age in Britain with socio-economic position: baseline data from a randomised controlled trial, *Journal of Epidemiology and Community Health*, 58: 667–73.

Brickman, P. and Bulman, R.J. (1977) Pleasure and pain in social comparison, in J.M. Suls and R.L. Miller (eds) *Social Comparison Processes: Theoretical and Empirical Perspectives*. Washington, DC: Hemisphere.

Brickman, P. and Campbell, D.T. (1971) *Hedonic Relativism and Planning the Good Society*, in M.H. Appley (ed.) *Adaptation-level Theory: A Symposium*. New York: Academic Press.

Bridgwood, A. (2000) *People Aged 65 and Over: Results of an Independent Study Carried out on Behalf of the Department of Health as part of the 1988 General Household Survey*. London: Office for National Statistics.

Bridgwood, A., Lilly, R., Thomas, M. et al. (2000) *Living in Britain: Results from the 1998 General Household Survey*. London: The Stationery Office.

Brissette, I., Cohen, S. and Seeman, T.E. (2000) Measuring social integration and social networks, in S. Cohen, L.G. Underwood and B.H. Gottlieb (eds) *Social Support Measurement and Intervention: A Guide for Health and Social Scientists*. Oxford: Oxford University Press.

Brouwer, A. (1990) The nature of ageing, in M.A. Horan and A. Brouwer (eds) *Gerontology: Approaches to Biomedical and Clinical Research*. London: Arnold.

Brown, G.W. and Harris, T. (1978) *Social Origins of Depression: A Study in Psychiatric Disorders in Women*. London: Tavistock.

Brown, J., Bowling, A. and Flyn, T. (2004) *Models of Quality of Life: a Taxonomy, Overview and Systematic Review of Quality of Life*. Sheffield: Department of Sociological Studies, European Forum on Population Ageing Research.

Browne, J.P., O'Boyle, C.A., McGee, H.M. *et al.* (1994) Individual quality of life in the healthy elderly, *Quality of Life Research*, 3: 235–44.

Browning, R. ([1864] 1979) Rabbi Ben Ezra, in J.F. Loucks (ed.) *Robert Browning's Poetry*. New York: W.W. Norton.

Bryant, L.L., Corbett, K.K. and Kutner, J.S. (2001) In their own words: a model of healthy ageing, *Social Science and Medicine*, 53: 927–41.

Burgess, E. (1960) *Aging in Western Societies*. Chicago: University of Chicago Press.

Burholt, V. (2001) *Ageing Well: A European Study of Adult Well-being*. Bangor: University of Wales.

Butt, D.S. and Beiser, M. (1987) Successful aging: a theme for international psychology, *Psychology and Aging*, 2: 87–94.

Buunk, B.P. and Gibbons, F.X. (1998) Social comparison in health and illness: a historical overview, in B.P. Bunk and F.X. Gibbons (eds) *Health, Coping and Well-being: Perspectives from Social Comparisons Theory*. Mahwah, NJ: Lawrence Erlbaum.

Calman, K.C. (1984) Quality of life in cancer patients – a hypothesis, *Journal of Medical Ethics*, 10: 124–7.

Campbell, A. (1972) Aspiration, satisfaction and fulfilment, in A. Campbell and P.E. Converse (eds) *The Human Meaning of Social Change*. New York: Sage.

Campbell, A. (1981) *The Sense of Well Being in America*. New York: McGraw-Hill.

Campbell, A., Converse, P. and Rogers, W.L. (1976) *The Quality of American Life: Perceptions, Evaluations and Satisfaction*. New York: Sage.

Cantril, H. (1967) *The Pattern of Human Concerns*. Camden, NJ: Rutgers University Press.

Caplan, G. (1974) *Support Systems and Community Mental Health*. New York: Behavioral Publications.

Carp, F.M. and Carp, A. (1981) Mental health characteristics and acceptance-rejection of old age, *American Journal of Orthopsychiatry*, 51: 230–41.

Carver, C.S. and Scheier, M.F. (1981) *Attention and Self-regulation: A Control-theory Approach to Human Behavior*. New York: Springer.

Carver, D.J., Chapman, C.A., Salazar, T. *et al.* (1999) Validity and reliability of the Medical Outcomes Study Short Form-20 questionnaire as a measure of quality of life in elderly people living at home, *Age and Ageing*, 28: 169–74.

Cassel, J. (1976) The contribution of the social environment to host resistance, *American Journal of Epidemiology*, 104: 107–23.

Cella, D.F. and Tulsky, D.S. (1990) Measuring quality of life today: methodological aspects, *Oncology*, 4: 29–38.

Clark, A.E. and Oswald, A.J. (1996) Satisfaction and comparison income, *Journal of Public Economics*, 61: 359–81.

Clark, M. and Andersson, B.G. (1967) *Culture and Aging: An Anthropological Study of Older Americans*. Springfield, IL: Charles C. Thomas.

Clark, P. and Bowling, A. (1989) Observational study of quality of life in NHS nursing homes and a long stay ward for the elderly, *Ageing and Society*, 9: 123–48.

Clark, P. and Bowling, A. (1990) Quality of everyday life in long stay institutions for the elderly: an observational study of long stay hospital and nursing home care, *Social Science and Medicine*, 30: 1201–10.

Clarke, L. and Roberts, C. (2004) The meaning of grandparenthood and its contribution to the quality of life of older people, in A. Walker (ed.) *Growing Older: Quality of Life in Old Age*. Maidenhead: Open University Press.

Clarke, P.J., Marshall, V.W., Ryff, C.D. and Rosenthal, C.J. (2000) Well-being in Canadian seniors: findings from the Canadian study of health and aging, *Canadian Journal on Aging*, 19: 139–59.

Cobb, S. (1976) Social support as a moderator of life stress, *Psychosomatic Medicine*, 38: 300–14.

Coleman, P. (1984) Assessing self-esteem and its sources in elderly people, *Ageing and Society*, 4: 117–35.

Coleman, P.G., McKiernan, F., Mills, M. and Speck, P. (2002) Spiritual belief and quality of life: the experience of older bereaved spouses, *Quality in Ageing – Policy, Practice and Research*, 3: 20–6.

Colman, J.S. (1988) Social capital in the creation of human capital, *American Journal of Sociology*, 94: S95–120.

Cooper, K., Arber, S., Fee, L. and Ginn, J. (1999) *The Influence of Social Support and Social Capital on Health: A Review and Analysis of British Data*. London: Health Education Authority..

Coopersmith, S. (1967) *The Antecedents of Self-esteem*. San Francisco: W.H. Freeman.

Costa, P.T. and McCrae, R.R. (1984) Personality as a lifelong determinant of well-being, in C. Lalatesta and C. Izard (eds) *Affective Processes in Adult Development and Aging*. Beverly Hills, CA: Sage.

Costa, P.T., Zonderman, A.B., McRae, R.R. *et al.* (1987) Longitudinal analysis of psychological well-being in national samples: stability of mean levels, *Journal of Gerontology*, 42: 50–5.

Cotton, S.R. (1999) Marital status and mental health revisited: examining the importance of risk factors and resources. *Journal of Applied Family Studies*, 48: 225–33.

Coulthard, M., Walker, A. and Morgan, A. (2001) *People's Perceptions of Their Neighbourhood and Community Involvement*. London: The Stationery Office.

Cramer, V., Torgersen, S. and Kringlen, E. (2004) Quality of life in the city: the effect of population density, *Social Indicators Research*, 69: 103–16.

Craven, P. and Wellman, B. (1974) The network city, in M.P. Effrat (ed.) *The Community: Approaches and Applications*. New York: Free Press.

Crawford, M. (1972) Retirement and role playing, *Sociology*, 6: 217–36.

Cumming, E. and Henry, E. (1961) *Growing Old: The Process of Disengagement*. New York: Basic Books.

Cummins, R.A. (2000) Objective and subjective quality of life: an interactive model, *Social Indicators Research*, in press.

242

Darnton-Hill, I. (1995) Healthy ageing and the quality of life, *World Health Forum*, 16: 335–43.

Davidson, K., Arber, S., Perren, K. and Daly, T. (2002) *Older Men: Partnership Status and Social Organisations*, paper presented at ESRC Growing Older programme meeting, London, 22 October.

Day, A.T. (1991) *Remarkable Survivors*. Washington, DC: Urban Institute Press.

De Vellis, R.F., Blalock, S.J., Holt, K. *et al.* (1990) The relationship of social comparison to rheumatoid arthritis symptoms and affect, *Basic and Applied Social Psychology*, 11: 1–18.

Delhey, J., Böhnke, P., Habich, R. and Zapf, W. (2002) Quality of life in a European perspective: the EUROMODULE as a new instrument for comparative welfare research, *Social Indicators Research*, 58: 163–76.

Department for Environment, Food and Rural Affairs (2002) *Quality of Life Barometer*. London: DEFRA.

Department of Transport (2000) *Older People: Their Transport Needs and Requirements*. London: Department of Transport.

Descartes, R. ([1637] 1953) *Discours de la Méthode: Sixiéme Partie*, in A. Bridoux (ed.) Descartes: Kuvres et Lettres. Paris: Gallimard.

Devins, G.M. and Seland, T.P. (1987) Emotional impact of multiple sclerosis: recent findings and suggestions for future research, *Psychological Bulletin*, 101: 363–75.

Diener, E. and Biswas-Myers, R. (2002) Will money increase subjective well-being? *Social Indicators Research*, 57: 119–69.

Diener, E. and Lucas, R.E. (2000) Subjective emotional well being, in M. Lewis and J.M. Haviland (eds) *Handbook of Emotions*, 2nd edn. New York: Guilford.

Diener, E. and Suh, E. (1997) Measuring quality of life: economic, social and subjective indicators. *Social Indicators Research*, 40: 189–216.

Diener, E., Emmons, R.A., Larson, R.J. and Griffin, S. (1985) The satisfaction with life scale, *Journal of Personality Assessment*, 49: 71–5.

Diener, E., Sandvik, E., Pavot, W. and Gallagher, D. (1991) Response artefacts in the measurement of subjective well-being, *Social Indicators Research*, 24: 35–56.

Dodd, T., Nicholas, S., Povey, D. and Walker, A. (2004) *Crime in England and Wales 2003/2004*. London: The Home Office.

Donald, C.A., Ware, J.E, Brook, R.H. *et al.* (1978) *Conceptualization and Measurement of Health for Adults in the Health Insurance Study*, vol. IV. Santa Monica, CA: Rand Corporation.

Dowd, J. (1975) Ageing as exchange: a preface to theory. *Journal of Gerontology*, 30: 584–94.

Doyal, L. and Gough, I. (1991) *A Theory of Human Need*. London: Macmillan.

Dubos, R. (1959) *Mirage of Health*. New York: Harper.

Dunnell, K. and Dix, D. (2000) Are we looking forward to a longer and healthier retirement? *Health Statistic Quarterly*, 6: 18–24.

Dupuy, H.J. (1984) The psychological general well-being index, in N.K. Wenger, M.E. Mattson, C.D. Furberg *et al.* (eds) *Assessment of Quality of Life in Clinical Trials of Cardiovascular Therapies.* New York: Le Jacq.

Durkheim, E. (1895) *The Rules of Sociological Method.* New York: Free Press [reprinted 1982].

Durkheim, E. (1897) *Suicide: A Study in Sociology.* New York: Free Press [reprinted 1997].

Easterlin, R.A. (1974) Does economic growth improve the human lot? Some empirical evidence, in P.A. David and M.W. Reder (eds) *Nations and Households in Economic Growth: Essays in Honor of Moses Abramowitz.* New York: Academic Press.

Easterlin, R.A. (1995) Will raising the incomes of all increase the happiness of all? *Journal of Economic Behavior and Organization*, 27: 35–47.

Ebrahim, S., Wannamethee, S.G., Whincup, P. *et al.* (2000) Locomotor disability in a cohort of British men: the impact of lifestyle and disease, *International Journal of Epidemiology*, 29: 478–86.

Eckenrode, J. and Hamilton, S. (2000) One-to-one support interventions, in S. Cohen, L.G. Underwood and B.H. Gottlieb (eds) *Social Support Measurement and Interventions: A Guide for Health and Social Scientists.* Oxford: Oxford University Press.

Economist Intelligence Unit (2004) *The World in 2005.* London: Economist Intelligence Unit.

Ehrhardt, J.J., Saris, W.E. and Veenhoven, R. (2000) Stability of life satisfaction over time: analysis of change in ranks in a national population, *Journal of Happiness Studies*, 1: 177–205.

Ekerdt, D.J. (1986) The busy ethic: moral continuity between work and retirement, *The Gerontologist*, 26: 239–44.

Emler, N. (2001) *Self-esteem.* York: Joseph Rowntree Foundation.

Engel, G.L. (1968) A life-setting conducive to illness: the giving up-given up complex, *Annals of Internal Medicine*, 69: 293–9.

Erikson, R. (1993) Descriptions of inequality: the Swedish approach to welfare research, in M. Nussbaum and A. Sen (eds) *The Quality of Life.* Oxford: Oxford University Press.

EuroQol Group (1990) EuroQol – a new facility for the measurement of health related quality of life, *Health Policy*, 16: 199–208.

Fabrigoule, C., Luc-Letenneuer, J.F.D., Mounir-Zarrouk, D. *et al.* (1995) Social and leisure activities and risk of dementia: a prospective longitudinal study, *Journal of the American Geriatrics Society*, 43: 485–90.

Falaschetti, E., Malbut, K. and Primatesta, P. (2002) *The General Health of Older People and Their Use of Health Services.* London: The Stationery Office.

Farquhar, M. (1995) Elderly people's definitions of quality of life, *Social Science and Medicine*, 41: 1439–46.

Fayers, P.M. and Hand, D.J. (2002) Causal variables, indicator variables and measurement scales: an example from quality of life, *Journal of the Royal Statistical Association*, 165(2): 1–21.

Feeny, D., Furlong, W., Boyle, M. and Torrance, G.W. (1995) Multi-attribute health status classification systems, Health Utilities Index, *Pharmaceconomics*, 7: 490–502.

Fennell, G., Phillipson, C. and Evers, H. (1988) *The Sociology of Old Age*. Milton Keynes: Open University Press.

Fernàndez-Ballesteros, R. (1993) The construct of quality of life among the elderly, in E. Beregi, A.A. Gergely and K. Rajczi (eds) *Recent Advances in Aging Science*. Bologna, Italy: Monduzzi Editore SpA.

Fernàndez-Ballesteros, R. (1998a) Quality of life: concept and assessment, in J.G. Adair, D. Bélanger and K.L. Dion (eds) *Advances in Psychological Science*. Hove: Psychology Press.

Fernàndez-Ballesteros, R. (1998b) Quality of life: the differential conditions, *Psychology in Spain*, 2: 57–65.

Fernàndez-Ballesteros, R. (2003) Light and dark in the psychology of human strengths: the example of psychogerontology, in L.G. Aspinwall and U.M. Saludinger (eds) *A Psychology of Human Strengths*. Washington, DC: American Psychological Association.

Festinger, L. (1954) A theory of social comparison processes, *Human Relations*, 7: 117–40.

Fisher, B.J. (1992) Successful aging and life satisfaction: a pilot study for conceptual clarification, *Journal of Aging Studies*, 6: 191–202.

Fisher, B.J. (1995) Successful aging: life satisfaction and generativity in later life, *International Journal of Aging and Human Development*, 41: 239–50.

Fisher, B.J. and Specht, D.K. (1999) Successful aging and creativity in later life, *Journal of Aging Studies*, 13: 457–72.

Fisher, B.J., Day, M. and Collier, C.E. (1992) Successful aging: volunteerism and generativity in later life, in D. Redburn and B. McNemara (eds) *Social Gerontology*. Westport, CT: Greenwood.

Fitts, W.H. (1965) *Tennessee Self-Concept Scale Manual*. Nashville, TN: Counselor Recordings and Tests.

Fitzgerald, T.E., Tennen, H., Affleck, G. and Pransky, G.S. (1993) The relative importance of dispositional optimism and control appraisals in quality of life after coronary bypass surgery, *Journal of Behavioral Medicine*, 16: 25–43.

Fitzpatrick, R. (1999) Assessment of quality of life as an outcome: finding measurements that reflect individual's priorities (editorial), *Quality in Health Care*, 8: 1–2.

Flax, M.J. (1972) *A Study in Comparative Urban Indicators: Conditions in 18 Large Metropolitan Areas*. Washington, DC: The Urban Institute.

Folkman, S. (1997) Positive psychological states and coping with severe stress, *Social Science and Medicine*, 45: 1207–21.

Fox-Rushby, J. and Parker, M. (1995) Culture and the measurement of health-related quality of life, *European Review of Applied Psychology*, 45: 257–63.

Freund, A.M. and Baltes, P.B. (1998) Selection, optimization, and compensation as strategies of life management: correlations with subjective indicators of successful aging, *Psychology and Aging*, 13: 531–43.

Freund, A.M. and Riediger, M. (2003) Successful aging, in R.M. Lerner (ed.) *Handbook of Psychology: Development Psychology*, vol. 6, pp. 601–28. New York: John Wiley and Sons.

Frey, B.S. and Stutzer, A. (2001) *Happiness and Economics*. Princeton, NJ: Princeton University Press.

Friedman, E. and Thomas, S.A. (1995) Pet ownership, social support and one-year survival after acute myocardial infarction in the cardiac arrhythmia suppression trial (CAST), *American Journal of Cardiology*, 76: 1213–17.

Fry, P.S. (2000) Whose quality of life is it anyway? Why not ask seniors to tell us about it? *International Journal of Aging and Human Development*, 50: 361–83.

Furnham, A. and Petrides, K.V. (2003) Trait emotional intelligence and happiness, *Social Behavior and Personality*, 31: 815–24.

Gabriel, Z. and Bowling, A. (2004a) Quality of life in older age from the perspectives of older people, in A. Walker and C. Hagen Hennessy (eds) *Growing Older: Quality of Life in Older Age*. Maidenhead: Open University Press.

Gabriel, Z. and Bowling, A. (2004b) Perspectives on quality of life in older age: older people talking, *Ageing and Society*, 24: 675–91.

Gardner, J. and Oswald, A. (2001) *Does Money Buy Happiness? A Longitudinal Study Using Data on Windfalls*. Warwick: University of Warwick, Department of Economics.

Garfein, A.J. and Herzog, A.R. (1995) Robust aging among the young-old, old-old and oldest-old, *Journal of Gerontology*, 50b: 577–87.

Garratt, A.M. and Ruta, D.A. (1999) The Patient-Generated Index, in C.R.B. Joyce, C.A. O'Boyle and H. McGee (eds) *Individual Quality of Life: Approaches to Conceptualisation and Assessment*. Amsterdam: Harwood Academic Publishers.

Garratt, A.M., Schmidt, L., Mackintosh, A. and Fitzpatrick, R. (2002) Quality of life measurement: bibliographic study of patient assessed health outcome measures, *British Medical Journal*, 324: 1417.

Gatz, M. and Zarit, S. (1999) A good old age: paradox or possibility, in V. Bengtson, J. Ruth and K. Schaie (eds) *Theories of Gerontology*. New York: Springer.

Gecas, V. (1989) The social psychology of self-efficacy, *Annual Review of Sociology*, 15: 291–316.

George, L.K. (1979) The happiness syndrome: methodological and substantive issues in the study of psychological well-being in adulthood, *Gerontologist*, 19: 210–16.

George, L.K., Blazer, D.G., Hughes, D.C. *et al.* (1989) Social support and the outcome of major depression, *British Journal of Psychiatry*, 154: 478–85.

Gibson, R.C. (1995) Promoting successful and productive aging in minority populations, in L.A. Bond, S.J. Cutler and A. Grams (eds) *Promoting Successful and Productive Aging*. London: Sage.

Gilhooley, M., Hamilton, K., O'Neill, M. *et al.* (2003) *Transport and Ageing: Extending Quality of Life via Public and Private Transport*. Sheffield: Growing Older Programme, University of Sheffield.

Gingold, R. (1999) *Successful Ageing*, 2nd edn. Oxford: Oxford University Press.

Gitlin, L.N. (2003) Conducting research on home environments: lessons learned and new directions, *The Gerontologist*, 43: 628–37.

Glass, T.A., Mendes de Leon, C., Marottoli, R.A. and Berkman, L.F. (1999) Population based study of social and productive activities as predictors of survival among elderly Americans, *British Medical Journal*, 319: 478–83.

Goddard, E. (1990) Measuring morbidity and some of the factors associated with it, in *Health and Lifestyle Surveys: Towards a Common Approach: Report of a Workshop Held on 7 November 1989 Organised by the HEA and OPCS*. London: HEA and OPCS.

Golant, S.M. (2003) Conceptualizing time and behavior in environmental gerontology: a pair of old issues deserving new thought, *The Gerontologist*, 43: 638–48.

Goldberg, D.P. and Williams, P. (1988) *A User's Guide to the General Health Questionnaire*. Windsor: NFER-Nelson.

Goldstein, M.S., Siegel, J.M. and Boyer, R. (1984) Predicting changes in perceived health status, *American Journal of Public Health*, 74: 611–15.

Goodchild, M.E. and Duncan Jones, P. (1985) Chronicity and the General Health Questionnaire, *British Journal of Psychiatry*, 146: 55–61.

Greig, C. (2002) The trainability of elderly people, *Age and Ageing*, 31: 223–4.

Grundy, E. (1997) The health of older adults 1841–1994, in J. Charlton and M. Murphy (eds) *The Health of Adult Britain 1841–1994*, vol. II. London: The Stationery Office.

Grundy, E. (2001) Ageing and vulnerable elderly people in Europe, paper prepared for NIEPS (Network for Integrated European Population Studies) workshop, Rome, April 2001.

Grundy, E. and Bowling, A. (1997) The sociology of ageing, in R. Jacoby and C. Oppenheimer (eds) *Psychiatry in the Elderly*, 2nd edn. Oxford: Oxford University Press.

Grundy, E. and Bowling, A. (1999) Enhancing the quality of extended life years: identification of the oldest old with a very good and very poor quality of life, *Ageing and Mental Health*, 3: 199–212.

Grundy, E. and Holt, G. (2001) The socio-economic status of older adults: how should we measure it in studies of health inequalities? *Journal of Epidemiology and Community Health*, 55: 895–904.

Grundy, E., Bowling, A. and Farquhar, M. (1996) Social support, life satisfaction and survival at older ages, in G. Casselli and A. Lopez (eds) *Health and Mortality Among Elderly Populations*. Oxford: Clarendon Press.

Guillemard, A.M. (1982) Old age, retirement and the social class structure: toward an analysis of the structural dynamics of the later stage of life, in T.K. Hareven and K.J. Adams (eds) *Ageing and Life Course Transitions: An Interdisciplinary Perspective*. London: Tavistock.

Gurin, G., Verloff, J. and Field, S. (1960) *Americans View Their Mental Health*. New York: Basic Books.

Hagerty, M.R., Cummins, R., Ferriss, A.L. *et al.* (2001) Quality of life indexes for national policy: review and agenda for research, *Social Indicators Research*, 55: 1–96.

Hagerty, M.R., Vogel, J. and Miller, V. (eds) (2004) *Assessing Quality of Life and Living Conditions to Guide National Policy*. Netherlands: Kluwer.

Harkin, J. and Huber, J. (2004) *Eternal Youths: How the Baby Boomers are Having their Time Again*. London: DEMOS.

Hartman-Stein, P.E. and Potkanowicz, E.S. (2003) Behavioral determinants of healthy aging: good news for the baby boomer generation, *Online Journal of Issues in Nursing*, 8: 6.

Haug, M.R. and Folmar, S.J. (1986) Longevity, gender and life quality, *Journal of Health and Social Behavior*, 27: 332–45.

Havighurst, R.J. (1963) Successful aging, in R.H. Williams, C. Tibbits and W. Donahue (eds) *Processes of Aging*, vol. 1. New York: Atherton Press.

Havighurst, R.J. and Albrecht, R. (1953) *Older People*. New York: Longmans Green.

Havighurst, R.L., Neugarten, B. and Tobin, S.S. (1968) Disengagement and patterns of aging, in B.L. Neugarten (ed.) *Middle Age and Aging: A Reader in Social Psychology*. Chicago: University of Chicago Press.

Hayden, C., Boaz, A. and Taylor, F. (1999) *Attitudes and Aspirations of Older People: A Qualitative Study*. Warwick: Warwick Business School on behalf of Department of Social Security.

Hayes, R.D. and Ross, C.E. (1986) Body and mind: the effect of exercise, overweight, and physical health on psychological well-being, *Journal of Health and Social Behavior*, 27: 387–400.

Headey, B.W. and Wearing, A. (1989) Personality, life events, and subjective well-being: toward a dynamic equilibrium model, *Journal of Personality and Social Psychology*, 57: 1–9.

Headey, B.W. and Wearing, A. (1992) *Understanding Happiness: A Theory of Subjective Well-being*. Melbourne: Longman.

Headey, B.W., Glowacki, T., Holmstrom, E.L. and Wearing, A.J. (1985) Modelling change in perceived quality of life, *Social Indicators Research*, 17: 276–98.

Heidrich, S.M. and Ryff, C.D. (1993a) Physical and mental health in later life: the self-esteem as mediator, *Psychology and Aging*, 8: 327–38.

Heidrich, S.M. and Ryff, C.D. (1993b) The role of social comparisons processes in the psychological adaptation of elderly adults, *Journal of Gerontology*, 48: 127–36.

Heidrich, S.M. and Ryff, C.D. (1995) Health, social comparisons and psychological well-being: their cross-time relationships, *Journal of Adult Development*, 2: 173–86.

Hemingway, H. and Marmot, M. (1999) Psychosocial factors in the aetiology and prognosis of coronary heart disease: systematic review of prospective cohort studies, *British Medical Journal*, 318: 1460–7.

Heylighten, F. and Bernheim, J. (2000) Global progress I: empirical evidence for ongoing increase in quality of life, *Journal of Happiness Studies*, I: 323–49.

Hickey, A., O'Boyle, C.A,. McGee, H.M. and Joyce, C.R.B. (1999) The schedule for the evaluation of individual quality of life, in C.R.B. Joyce, C.A. O'Boyle and H. McGee (eds) *Individual Quality of Life: Approaches to Conceptualisation and Assessment.* Amsterdam: Harwood Academic Publishers.

Higgs, P., Hyde, M., Wiggins, R. and Blane, D. (2003) Researching quality of life in early old age: the importance of the sociological dimension, *Social Policy and Administration*, 37: 239–52.

Hill, C., Edwards, G., Myers, C. *et al.* (1999) *Social Focus on Older People.* London: Office for National Statistics.

Holahan, J.C. and Moos, R.H. (1981) Social support and psychological distress: a longitudinal analysis, *Journal of Abnormal Psychology*, 90: 365–70.

Home Office (2000) *Recorded Crime Statistics*, 1999–2000. London: Home Office.

Hooper, D. and Ineichen, B. (1979) Adjustment to moving: a follow-up study of the mental health of young families in new housing, *Social Science and Medicine*, 13D: 163–8.

Hörnquist, J.O. (1982) The concept of quality of life, *Scandinavian Journal of Social Medicine*, 10: 57–61.

House, J.S. (1981) *Work, Stress and Social Support.* Reading, MA: Addison-Wesley.

House, J.S., Landis, K.R. and Umberson, D. (1988) Social relationships and health, *Science*, 241: 540–4.

House J.S., Lepkowski, J.M., Kinney, A.M. *et al.* (1994) The social stratification of aging and health, *Journal of Health and Social Behavior*, 35: 213–34.

Hudler, M. and Richter, R. (2002) Cross-national comparison of the quality of life in Europe: inventory of surveys and methods, *Social Indicators Research*, 58: 217–28.

Huber, J. and Skidmore, P. (2003) *The New Old: Why the Baby Boomers Won't Be Pensioned Off.* London: DEMOS.

Hughes, B. (1990) Quality of life, in S.M. Peace (ed.) *Researching Social Gerontology.* London: Sage.

Hughes, S.L., Giobbie-Hurder, A., Weaver, F.M. *et al.* (1999) Relationship between caregiver burden and health-related quality of life, *Gerontologist*, 39: 534–45.

Huisman, M., Kunst, A.E., Andersen, O. *et al.* (2004) Socio-economic inequalities in mortality among the elderly in eleven European populations, *Journal of Epidemiology and Community Health*, 58: 468–75.

Hyde, M., Wiggins, R.D., Higgs, P. and Blane, D.B. (2003) A measure of quality of life in early old age: the theory, development and properties of a needs satisfaction model (CASP-19), *Ageing and Mental Health*, 7: 186–94.

Hyman, H. (1942) The psychology of subjective status, *Psychological Bulletin*, 39: 473–4.

Hyppa, M.T. and Maki, J. (2003) Social participation and health in a community rich in stock of social capital, *Health Education Research*, 18: 770–9.

Idler, E.I. and Kasl, S.V. (1995) Self-ratings of health: do they also predict change in functional ability? *Journal of Gerontology* (B), 50: S344–53.

Idler, E.L. and Benyamini, Y. (1997) Self-rated health and mortality: a review of twenty-seven community studies, *Journal of Health and Social Behavior*, 38: 21–37.

Inglehart, R. and Rabier, J.R. (1986) Aspirations adapt to situations – but why are the Belgians so much happier than the French? A cross-cultural analysis of the subjective quality of life, in F.M. Andrews (ed.) *Research on the Quality of Life*. Survey Research Center, Institute for Social Research University of Michigan.

Iwarsson, S. (2003) Assessing the fit between older people and their home environments – an occupational therapy research perspective, in H.W. Wahl, R. Scheidt and P. Windley (eds) *Annual Review of Gerontology and Geriatrics: Ageing in Context: Socio-physical Environments*, vol. 23. New York: Springer.

James, O. (1997) *Britain on the Couch*. London: Century.

James, O. (2003) *They F*** You Up*. London: Bloomsbury.

Jaracz, K., Gustafsson, G. and Hamrin, E. (2004) The life situation and functional capacity of the elderly with locomotor disability in Sweden and Poland according to a model by Lawton, *International Journal of Nursing Practice*, 10: 45–53.

Jenkinson, C., Ziebland, S., Fitzpatrick, R. *et al.* (1991) Sensitivity to change of weighted and unweighted versions of two health status measures, *International Journal of Health Sciences*, 2: 189–94.

Johansson, S. (2002) Conceptualising and measuring quality of life for national policy: from the Swedish Level of Living Survey to an epistemology of the democratic process, *Social Indicators Research*, 58: 13–32.

Johnson, C.J. (1983) Dyadic family elations and social support, *The Gerontologist*, 23: 377–83.

Joyce, C.R.B., McGee, H.M. and O'Boyle, C.A. (1999) Individual quality of life: review and outlook, in C.R.B. Joyce, C.A. O'Boyle and H. McGee (eds) *Individual Quality of Life: Approaches to Conceptualisation and Assessment*. Amsterdam: Harwood Academic Publishers.

Juniper, E.F., Guyatt, G.H., Ferrie, P.J. and Griffith, L.E. (1993) Measuring quality of life in asthma, *American Review of Respiratory Disease*, 147: 832–8.

Juniper, E.F., Guyatt, G.H., Streiner, D.L. and King, D.R. (1997) Clinical impact versus factor analysis for quality of life questionnaire construction, *Journal of Clinical Epidemiology*, 50: 233–8.

Jylhä, M. (2001) Old age and loneliness – cross-sectional and longitudinal analyses in the Tampere longitudinal study on aging, paper presented at the International Congress of Gerontology, Vancouver, July.

Kahana, E., Lovegreen, L., Kahana, B. and Kahana, M. (2003) Person, environment, and person-environment fit as influences on residential satisfaction of elders, *Environment and Behavior*, 35: 434–53.

Kane, R.L, Rockwood, T., Philp, I. and Finch, M. (1998) Differences in valuation of functional status components among consumers and professionals in Europe and the United States, *Journal of Clinical Epidemiology*, 51: 657–66.

Kaplan, B.H. (1975) An epilogue: toward further research on family and health, in B.H. Kaplan and J.C. Cassel (eds) *Family and Health: An Epidemiological Approach*. Chapel Hill, NC: University of North Carolina, Institute for Research and Social Science.

Kaplan, G.A. and Camacho, T. (1983) Perceived health and mortality: a nine-year follow-up of the Human Population Laboratory Cohort, *American Journal of Epidemiology*, 117: 292–8.

Kaplan, B.H., Cassel, J.C. and Gore, S. (1977) Social support and health, *Medical Care*, 15: 47–58.

Kaplan, G.A., Strawbridge, W.J. and Camacho, T. *et al.* (1993) Factors associated with change in physical functioning in the elderly: a six year prospective study, *Journal of Aging and Health*, 5: 140–53.

Kaplan, G.A., Strawbridge, W.J., Cohen, R.D. and Hungerford, L.R. (1996) Natural history of leisure time: physical activity and its correlates: associations with mortality from all causes and cardiovascular disease over 28 years, *American Journal of Epidemiology*, 144: 793–7.

Kasser, T. (2002) *The High Price of Materialism*. Cambridge, MA: MIT Press.

Katz, M.H. (1999) *Multivariable Analysis: A Practical Guide for Clinicians*. Cambridge: Cambridge University Press.

Kawachi, I. and Berkman, L. (2000) Social cohesion, social capital and health, in L.F. Berkman and I. Kawachi (eds) *Social Epidemiology*. Oxford: Oxford University Press.

Kawachi, I., Kennedy, B.P., Lochner, K. and Prothrow-Stith, D. (1997a) Social capital, income inequality and mortality, *American Journal of Public Health*, 87: 1491–8.

Kawachi, I., Kennedy, B.P. and Lochner, K. (1997b) Long live community: social capital as public health, *American Prospect*, Nov/Dec: 56–9.

Kawachi, I., Kennedy, B.P. and Glass, R. (1999) Social capital and self-rated health: a contextual analysis, *American Journal of Public Health*, 89: 1187–93.

Kellaher, L., Peace, S.M. and Holland, C. (2004) Environment, identity and old age – quality of life or a life of quality, in A. Walker and C. Hagen Hennessy (eds) *Growing Older: Quality of Life in Older Age*. Maidenhead: Open University Press.

Kelly, S. and Baker, A. (2000) Healthy life expectancy in Britain, 1980–96, and its use as an indicator in United Kingdom Government strategies, *Health Statistics Quarterly*, 7: 32–7.

Kendig, H. (2003) Directions in environmental gerontology: a multidisciplinary field, *The Gerontologist*, 43: 611–14.

Khaw, K.T. (1997) Healthy ageing, *British Medical Journal*, 315: 1090–6.

Kling, K.C., Ryff, C.D. and Essex, M.J. (1997) Adaptive changes in the self-concept during a life transition, *Personality and Social Psychology Bulletin*, 23: 989–98.

Koch, T. (2000) The illusion of paradox: commentary on 'Albrecht, G.L. and Devlieger, P.J. (1998) The disability paradox: high quality of life against all odds', *Social Science and Medicine*, 50: 757–9.

Koenig, H.G. (1995) Religion and health in later life, in M.A. Kimble, S.H. McFadden, J.W. Ellor and J.J. Seeber (eds) *Aging, Spirituality, and Religion: A Handbook*. Minneapolis, MN: Fortress Press.

Kogevinas, M., Marmot, M.G., Fox, A.J. *et al.* (1991) Socio-economic differences in cancer survival, *Journal of Epidemiology and Community Health*, 45: 216–19.

Kozma, A., Stones, M.J. and McNeil, J.K. (1991) *Subjective Well-being in Later Life*. Toronto: Butterworths.

Krupinski, J. (1980) Health and quality of life, *Social Science and Medicine*, 14A: 203–11.

Kushman, J. and Lane, S. (1980) A multi-variate analysis of factors affecting perceived life satisfaction and psychological well-being among the elderly, *Social Science Quarterly*, 61: 264–77.

Kutner, B., Fansel, D., Togo, A.M. *et al.* (1956) *Five Hundred Over 60*. New York: Sage.

Laing & Buisson (2004) *Care of Elderly People: Market Survey 2000*, 17th edn. London: Laing & Buisson.

Larson, R. (1978) Thirty years of research on the subjective well-being of older Americans, *Journal of Gerontology*, 33: 109–25.

Lau, R.R., Hartman, K.A. and Ware, J.E. (1986) Health as a value: methodological and theoretical considerations, *Health Psychology*, 5: 25–43.

Lawton, M.P. (1972) The dimensions of morale, in D. Kent, R. Kastenbaum and S. Sherwood (eds) *Research, Planning and Action for the Elderly*. New York: Behavioral Publications.

Lawton, M.P. (1975) The Philadelphia Geriatric Morale Scale: a revision, *Journal of Gerontology*, 30: 85–9.

Lawton, M.P. (1980) *Environment and Aging*. Monterrey, CA: Brooks Cole.

Lawton, M.P. (1982) Competence, environmental press and adaptation of older people, in M.P. Lawton, P.G. Windley and T.O. Byerts (eds) *Aging and Environment: Theoretical Approaches*. New York: Springer.

Lawton, M.P. (1983a) Environment and other determinants of well-being in older people, *Gerontologist*, 23: 349–57.

Lawton, M.P. (1983b) The varieties of wellbeing, *Experimental Aging Research*, 9: 65–72.

Lawton, M.P. (1991) Background: a multi-dimensional view of quality of life in frail elders, in J.E. Birren, J. Lubben, J. Rowe and D. Deutchman (eds) *The Concept and Measurement of Quality of Life in the Frail Elderly*. San Diego, CA: Academic Press.

Lawton, M.P. (1996) Quality of life and affect in later life, in C. Magai and S.H. McFadden (eds) *Handbook on Emotion, Human Development, and Aging*. San Diego, CA: Academic Press.

Lawton, M.P. and Nahemow, L. (1973) Ecology and the aging process, in C. Eisdorfer and M.P. Lawton (eds) *Psychology of Adult Development and Aging*. Washington, DC: American Psychological Association.

Lefcourt, H.M. (1982) *Locus of Control: Current Trends in Theory and Research*. Hillsdale, NJ: Lawrence Erlbaum.

Lehman, A.F. (1983) The well-being of chronic mental patients: assessing their quality of life, *Archives of General Psychiatry*, 40: 369–73.

Lehman, A.F. (1988) A quality of life interview for the chronically mentally ill, *Evaluation and Program Planning*, 11: 51–62.

Lemon, B., Bengtson, V. and Peterson, J. (1972) An exploration of the activity theory of aging: activity types and life satisfaction among in-movers to a retirement community, *Journal of Gerontology*, 27: 511–23.

Levi, P. (1958) *If this is a Man*, trans S. Woolf. London: Abacus.

Liberman, M.A. (1991) Relocation of the frail elderly, in J.E. Birren, J.E. Lubben, J.C. Rowe and D.E. Deutchman (eds) *The Concept and Measurement of Quality of Life in the Frail Elderly*. San Diego, CA: Academic Press.

Lindeström, M. (2004) Social capital, the miniaturisation of community and self-reported global and psychological health, *Social Science and Medicine*, 59: 595–607.

Logan, J.R., Ward, R. and Spitze, G. (1992) As old as you feel: age identity in middle and later life, *Social Forces*, 71: 451–67.

Lowenthal, M.F. and Haven, C. (1968) Interaction and adaptation: intimacy as a critical variable, *American Sociology Review*, 33: 20–30.

Lykken, D. and Tellegen, A. (1996) Happiness is a stochastic phenomenon, *Psychological Science*, 7: 186–9.

Machenbach, J.P., Kunst, A.E., Cavelaars, A.E. *et al.* (1997) Socioeconomic inequalities in morbidity and mortality in Western Europe, *Lancet*, 349: 1655–9.

Macintyre, S., Ellaway, A., Kearns, A. and Hiscock, R. (2000) *Housing Tenure and Car Ownership: Why Do They Predict Health and Longevity? Research Findings 7 – Economic and Social Research Council Health Variations Programme*. Lancaster: Department of Applied Social Science, Lancaster University.

Macleod, M.D. (1999) 'Why did it happen to me?' The role of social cognition processes in adjustment and recovery from criminal victimisation and illness, *Current Psychology*, 18: 18–31.

Maddox, G.L. (1963) Activity and morale: a longitudinal study of selected elderly subjects, *Social Forces*, 42: 195–204.

Malbut, K., Dinan, S. and Young, A. (2002) Aerobic training in the 'oldest old': the effect of 24 weeks of training, *Age and Ageing*, 31: 255–60.

Manton, K.G., Corder, L.S. and Stallard, E. (1993) Estimates of change in chronic disability and institutional incidence and prevalence rates in the US elderly population from the 1982, 1984 and 1989 National Long Term Care Survey, *Journal of Gerontology*, S48, S153–66.

Manton, K.G., Stallard, E. and Corder, L.S. (1995) Changes in co-morbidity and chronic disability in the US elderly population: evidence from the 1982, 1984 and 1989 National Long-term Care Survey, *Journal of Gerontology*, 50: S104–204.

Markides, K.S. and Martin, H.W. (1979) A causal model of life satisfaction among the elderly, *Journal of Gerontology*, 34: 86–93.

Markides, K.S. and Pappas, C. (1982) Subjective age, health and survivorship in old age, *Research on Aging*, 4: 87–96.

Marmot, M. (2004) *Status Syndrome*. London: Bloomsbury.

Marmot, M., Bosma, H., Hemingway, H. *et al.* (1997) Contribution of job control and other risk factors for social variations in coronary heart disease incidence: Whitehall II Study, *Lancet*, 350: 235–9.

Marmot, M., Banks, J., Blundell, R. *et al.* (eds) (2003) *Health, Wealth and Lifestyles of the Older Population in England: The 2002 English Longitudinal Study of Ageing*. London: Institute of Fiscal Studies.

Martin, J., Meltzer, H. and Elliot, D. (1988) *The Prevalence of Disability Among Adults: OPCS Surveys of Disability in Great Britain*, report no. 1. London: HMSO.

Maslow, A. (1954) *Motivation and Personality*. New York: Harper.

Maslow, A. (1968) *Toward a Psychology of Being*, 2nd edn. Princeton, NJ: Van Nostrand.

McKennell, A.C. (1978) Cognitive and affect in perceptions of well-being, *Social Indicators Research*, 5: 389–426.

McKevitt, C., Wolfe, C. and La Placa, V. (2002) *Comparing Professional and Patient Perspectives on Quality of Life*. ESRC Growing Older Programme: Research Findings, 2.

McMurdo, M. (2000) A healthy old age: realistic or futile goal? *British Medical Journal*, 32: 1149–51.

Mechanic, D. and Angel, R.J. (1987) Some factors associated with the report and evaluation of back pain, *Journal of Health and Social Behavior*, 28: 131–9.

Meeberg, G.A. (1993) Quality of life: a concept analysis, *Journal of Advanced Nursing*, 13: 32–8.

Menec, V.H. and Chipperfield, J.G. (1997) Remaining active in later life, the role of locos of control in senior's leisure activity participation, health and life satisfaction, *Journal of Ageing and Health*, 9: 105–25.

Mercer Human Resource Consulting (2003) *Mercer World-wide Quality of Life Survey: Personal Safety Rankings*. Geneva: Mercer Global Information Services.

Mercier, C. and King, S. (1993) A latent variable causal model of the quality of life and community tenure of psychotic patients, *Acta Psychiatrica Scandinavica*, 89: 72–7.

Michalos, A.C. (1985) Multiple discrepancies theory (MDT), *Social Indicators Research*, 16: 347–413.

Michalos, A.C. (1986) Job satisfaction, marital satisfaction and the quality of life: a review and preview, in F.M. Andrews (ed.) *Research on the Quality of Life*. Ann Arbor, MI: Survey Research Center, Institute for Social Research, University of Michigan.

Michalos, A.C. (1991) *Global Report on Student Well-being, Vol. 1: Life Satisfaction and Happiness*. New York: Springer-Verlag.

Michalos, A.C. and Zumbo, B.D. (2000) Criminal victimization and the quality of life, *Social Indicators Research*, 50: 245–95.

Michalos, A.C., Zumbo, B.D. and Hubley, A. (2000) Health and the quality of life, *Social Indicators Research*, 51: 245–86.

Michalos, A.C., Hubley, A.M., Zumbo, B.D. and Hemingway, D. (2001) Health and other aspects of the quality of life of older people, *Social Indicators Research*, 54: 239–74.

Mirowsky, J. and Ross, C.E. (1991) Eliminating defence and agreement bias from measures of the Sense of Control Index: a 2×2 index, *Social Psychology Quarterly*, 54: 127–45.

Mirowsky, J. and Ross, C.E. (1992) Age and depression, *Journal of Health and Social Behavior*, 33: 187–205.

Mitchell, J.C. (1969) The concept and use of social networks, in J.C. Mitchell (ed.) *Social Networks in Urban Situations: Analysis of Personal Relationships in Central African Towns*. Manchester: Manchester University Press.

Moen, P., Dempster-McClain, D. and Williams, R.M. (1989) Social integration and longevity: an event history analysis of women's roles and resilience, *American Sociological Review*, 54: 635–47.

Moriarty, D.G., Zack, M.M. and Kobau, R. (2003) The Centers for Disease Control and Prevention's Healthy Days measures – population tracking of perceived physical and mental health over time, *Health and Quality of Life Outcomes*, 1: 37.

Mroczek, D. and Kolarz, C. (1998) The effect of age on positive and negative affect: a developmental perspective on happiness, *Journal of Personality and Social Psychology*, 75: 1333–49.

Muntaner, C. and Lynch, J. (2002) Social capital, class gender, race conflict, and population health: an essay review of Bowling Alone's implications for social epidemiology, *International Journal of Epidemiology*, 31: 261–7.

Murray, J., Schneider, J., Banerjee, S. and Mann, A. (1999) Eurocare: a cross-national study of co-resident spouse carers for people with Alzheimer disease: II – a qualitative analysis of the experience of caregiving, *International Journal of Geriatric Psychiatry*, 14: 662–7.

Mutran, E. and Burke, P.J. (1979) Personalism as a component of old age identity, *Research on Aging*, 1: 37–64.

National Institute of Clinical Excellence (2005) *Scope Falls: Assessment and Prevention of Falls in Older People*. London: NICE.

Nazroo, J., Bajekal, M., Blane, D. and Grewal, I. (2004) Ethnic inequalities, in A. Walker and C. Hagan Hennessy (eds) *Growing Older: Quality of Life in Old Age*. Maidenhead: Open University Press.

Nelson, C., Murray, R., Henke, N. *et al.* (2001) Expectations of the 2020 UK health care system, in *Health Trends Review: Proceedings of a Conference Held by Her Majesty's Treasury Health Trends Review Team*. Barbican Conference Centre, London, 18 and 19 November. London: HM Treasury.

Netten, A., Smith, P., Healey, A. *et al.* (2002) *OPUS: A Measure of Social Care Outcome for Older People*. Canterbury: Personal Social Services Research Unit, University of Kent, PSSRU Research Summary no. 23.

Neugarten, B.L., Havighurst, R.J. and Tobin, S.S. (1961) The measurement of life satisfaction, *Journal of Gerontology*, 16: 134–43.

Neugarten, B., Havighurst, S. and Tobin, S. (1968) Personality and patterns of aging, in B. Neugarten (ed.) *Middle Age and Aging*. Chicago: University of Chicago Press.

New Philanthropy Capital (2004) *Grey Matters: Growing Older in Deprived Areas*. London: NPC.

Nilsson, M., Ekman, S.L and Sarvimäki, A. (1998) Ageing with joy or resigning to old age: older people's experiences of the quality of life in old age, *Health Care in Later Life*, 3: 94–110.

Noll, H.H. (2002a) Towards a European system of social indicators: theoretical framework and system architecture, *Social Indicators Research*, 58: 47–87.

Noll, H.H. (2002b) Social indicators and quality of life research: background, achievements and current trends, in N. Genov (ed.) *Advances in Sociological Knowledge Over Half a Century*. Paris: International Social Science Council.

Noll, H.H. and Zapf, W. (1994) Social indicators research: societal monitoring and social reporting, in I. Borg and P.P. Mohler (eds) *Trends and Perspectives in Empirical Social Research*. Berlin: Walter de Gruyer.

Nybo, H., Gaist, D., Jeune, B. *et al.* (2001) Functional status and self-rated health in 2,262 nonagenarians: the Danish 1905 cohort survey, *Journal of the American Geriatrics Society*, 49: 601–9.

Nydegger, C. (1986) Measuring morale and life satisfaction, in C.L. Fry and J. Keith (eds) *New Methods for Old Age Research: Strategies for Studying Diversity*. Boston, MA: Bergin and Garvey.

O'Boyle, C.A. (1997) Measuring the quality of later life, *Philosophy Transactions of the Royal Society of London*, 352: 1871–9.

Offer, A. (1997) Between the gift and the market: the economy of regard, *Economic History Review*, 50: 450–76.

Office for National Statistics (1999) The demography of centenarians in England and Wales, *Population Trends*, 96.

Office for National Statistics (2002) *Internet Access: Household and Individuals*, Release 24, www.statistics.gov.uk/releases.

Office for National Statistics (2003) *Census 2001: National Report for England and Wales*. London: The Stationery Office.

Office for National Statistics (2004) *Focus on Older People*. London: ONS.

Olsen, O. (1992) Impact of social network on cardiovascular mortality in middle-aged Danish men, *Journal of Epidemiology and Community Health*, 47: 176–80.

Olson, J.M. (1996) Resentment about deprivation: entitlement and hopefulness as mediators of the effects of qualifications, in J.M. Olson, C.P. Herman and M.P. Zanna (eds) *Relative Deprivation and Social Comparison: The Ontario Symposium*, vol. 4. Mahwah, NJ: Lawrence Erlbaum.

Ostir, G.V., Markides, K.S., Black, S.A. and Goodwin, J.S. (2000) Emotional well-being predicts subsequent functional independence and survival, *Journal of the American Geriatric Society*, 48: 473–8.

Ostir, G.V., Markides, K.S., Black, S.A. and Goodwin, J.S. (2001a) The association between emotional well-being and the incidence of stroke in older adults, *Psychosomatic Medicine*, 63: 210–15.

Ostir, G.V., Oeek, M.K., Markides, K.S. and Goodwin, J.S. (2001b) The association of emotional well-being on future risk of myocardial infarction in older adults, *Primary Psychiatry*, 8: 34–8.

Ostir, G.V., Ottenbacher, J.K. and Markides, K.S. (2004) Onset of frailty in older adults and the protective role of positive affect, *Psychology and Aging*, 19: 402–8.

Oswald, A.J. and Frank, R.H. (1997) Happiness and economic performance, *The Economic Journal*, 107: 1815–31.

Palmore, E.B. (1979) Predictors of successful aging, *The Gerontologist*, 19: 427–31.

Palmore, E.B. and Kivett, V. (1977) Changes in life satisfaction, *Journal of Gerontology*, 32: 311–16.

Palmore, E.B. and Luikart, C. (1972) Health and social factors related to life satisfaction, *Journal of Health and Social Behavior*, 13: 68–79.

Palmore, E.B., Nowlin, J.B. and Wang, H.S. (1985) Predictors of function among the old-old: a 10 year follow-up, *Journal of Gerontology*, 40: 244–50.

Parsons, T. (1951) *The Social System*. New York: Free Press.

Patrick, D.L. (2003) Patient-reported outcomes (PROs): an organising tool for concepts, measures, and applications, *Quality of Life Newsletter*, Fall: 1–5.

Patrick, D.L. and Erickson, P. (1993) *Health Status and Health Policy: Quality of Life in Health Care Evaluation and Resource Allocation*. New York: Oxford University Press.

Payne, B. (1988) Religious patterns and participation of older adults: a sociological perspective, *Educational Gerontology*, 14: 255–67.

Pearlin, L.I. (1989) The sociological study of stress, *Journal of Health and Social Behavior*, 30: 241–56.

Pearlin, L.I. (1999) Stress and mental health: a conceptual overview, in A.V. Horwitz and T.L. Scheid (eds) *Handbook for the Study of Mental Health: Social Contexts, Theories and Systems*. Cambridge: Cambridge University Press.

Pearlin, L.I. and Schooler, C. (1978) The structure of coping, *Journal of Health and Social Behavior*, 19: 2–21.

Peeters, A., Bouwman, G.D. and Knipscheer, C.P.M. (2001) *National Review on Quality of Life in Old Age*. Amsterdam: Vrije Universiteit Amsterdam, Institute for Applied Gerontology.

Perls, T.T. and Silver, M.H. (1999) *Living to 100: Lessons in Living to Your Maximum Potential at Any Age*. New York: Basic Books.

Péron, Y. (1992) A stage in the promotion of disability-free life expectancy as a health indicator, in J.M. Robine, M. Blanchet and J.E. Dowd (eds) *Health Expectancy: First*

Workshop of the International Healthy Life Expectancy Network (REVES) – Studies on Medical and Population Subjects, no. 54. London: HMSO.

Perrig-Chiello, P. (1999) Resources of well-being in elderly: differences between young old and old, in C. Hummel (ed.) *Les Sciences Sociales Face au Défi de la Grande Viellesse*. Geneva: Questions d'Age.

Pfizer (2002) *Pfizer Pan-European Healthy Ageing Survey*. Richmond: Taylor Nelson Sofres, Social Research Division.

Phelan, E.A., Anderson, L.A., Lacroix, A.Z. and Larson, E.B. (2004) Older adults' views of 'successful aging' – how do they compare with researchers' definitions? *Journal of the American Geriatrics Society*, 52: 211–16.

Phillipson, C. (1987) The transition to retirement, in G. Cohen (ed.) *Social Change in the Life Course*. London: Tavistock.

Pickett, K.E. and Pearl, M. (2001) Multilevel analyses of neighbourhood socioeconomic context and health outcomes: a critical review, *Journal of Epidemiology and Community Health*, 55: 111–22.

Pilkington, P. (2002) Social capital and health: measuring and understanding social capital at a local level could help to tackle health inequalities more effectively, *Journal of Public Health Medicine*, 24: 156–9.

Puner, M. (1974) *To the Good Long Life: What We Know About Growing Old*. London: Macmillan.

Putnam, M. (2002) Linking aging theory and disability models: increasing the potential to explore aging with physical impairment, *The Gerontologist*, 42: 799–806.

Putnam, R.D. (1995) Bowling alone: America's declining social capital, *Journal of Democracy*, 6: 65–78.

Putnam, R.D. (2000) *Bowling Alone: The Collapse and Revival of American Community*. New York: Simon & Schuster.

Qureshi, H., Nocon, A. and Thomson, C. (1994) *Measuring Outcomes of Community Care for Users and Carers: A Review*. York: Social Policy Research Unit, University of York.

Raina, P., Waltner, T.D., Bonnett, B. *et al.* (1999) Influence of companion animals on the physical and psychological health of older people: an analysis of a one-year longitudinal study, *Journal of the American Geriatrics Society*, 47: 323–9.

Ranzijn, R. and Luszcz, M. (2000) Measurement of subjective quality of life in elders, *International Journal of Ageing and Human Development*, 50: 263–78.

Research into Ageing (2004) *How to Thrive Past 55*. London: Research into Ageing.

Resnick, N.M. (1997) How should clinical care of the aged differ? *Lancet*, 350: 1157–8.

Rettig, K.D. and Leichtentritt, R.D. (1999) A general theory for perceptual indicators of family life quality, *Social Indicators Research*, 47: 307–42.

Riley, M.W., Johnson, M. and Foner, A. (1972) *Ageing and Society: A Sociology of Age Stratification*. New York: Sage.

Robert, S. and House, J.S. (1996) SES differentials in health by age and alternative indicators of SES, *Journal of Aging and Health*, 8: 359–88.

Rogerson, R.J. (1995) Environmental and health-related quality of life: conceptual and methodological similarities, *Social Science and Medicine*, 41: 1373–82.

Rogerson, R.J., Findlay, A.M., Coombes, M.G. and Morris, A. (1989a) Indicators of quality of life, *Environment and Planning*, 21: 1655–66.

Rogerson, R.J., Morris, A., Findlay, A. and Paddison, R. (1989b) *Quality of Life in Britain's Intermediate Cities*. Glasgow: Department of Geography, Quality of Life Group, University of Glasgow.

Roizen, M.F. (1999) *Real Age: Are You as Young as You Can Be?* London: Thorsons.

Roizen, M.F. and Stephenson, E.A. (2003) *Feel and Look Younger Fast.* London: Thorsons.

Roos, N.P. and Havens, B. (1991) Predictors of successful aging: a twelve year study of Manitoba elderly. *American Journal of Public Health*, 81: 63–8.

Rosenberg, M. (1965) *Society and the Adolescent Self Image.* Princeton, NJ: Princeton University Press.

Rosenfield, S. (1989) The effects of women's employment: personal control and sex differences, *Journal of Health and Social Behavior*, 30: 77–91.

Rosenfield, S. (1992) Factors contributing to the subjective quality of life of the chronically mentally ill, *Journal of Health and Social Behavior*, 33: 299–315.

Rosenwaike, I. (1985) *The Extreme Aged in America: A Portrait of an Expanding Population.* Westport, CT: Greenwood Press.

Ross, C.E. and Mirowsky, J. (2001) Neighbourhood disadvantage, disorder and health, *Journal of Health and Social Behavior*, 42: 258–76.

Roux, A.V.D., Borrell, L.N., Haan, M. *et al.* (2004) Neighbourhood environments and mortality in an elderly cohort: results from the cardiovascular health study, *Journal of Epidemiology and Community Health*, 58: 917–23.

Rowe, J.W. and Kahn, R.I. (1987) Human aging: usual and successful, *Science*, 237: 143–9.

Rowe, J.W. and Kahn, R.I. (1997) Successful aging, *The Gerontologist*, 37: 433–40.

Rowe, J.W. and Kahn, R.I. (1998) *Successful Aging.* New York: Pantheon.

Ruberman, W., Weinblatt, E., Goldberg, J.D. and Chaudary, B.S. (1984) Psychosocial influences on mortality after myocardial infarction, *New England Journal of Medicine*, 311: 552–9.

Rubinstein, R. and Parmelee, P. (1992) Attachment to place and the representations of the life course by the elderly, in I. Altman and S. Low (eds) *Place Attachment.* New York: Plenum Press.

Ryff, C.D. (1989a) Happiness is everything, or is it? Explorations on the meaning of psychological well-being, *Journal of Personality and Social Psychology*, 57: 1069–81.

Ryff, C.D. (1989b) Beyond Ponce de Leon and life satisfaction, *International Journal of Behavioral Development*, 12: 35–55.

Ryff, C.D. (1999) Psychology and aging, in W. Hazzard, J. Blass, W. Ettinger, J. Halter and J. Ouslander (eds) *Principles of Geriatric Medicine and Gerontology*, 4th edn. New York: McGraw-Hill.

Ryff, C.D. and Singer, B. (1996) Psychological well-being: meaning, measurement, and implications for psychotherapy research, *Psychotherapy Psychosomatics*, 65: 14–23.

Sanders, C., Egger, M., Donovan, J. and Frankel, S. (1998) Reporting on quality of life in randomised trials: bibliographic study, *British Medical Journal*, 317: 1191–4.

Saris, W.E. (1996) Integration of data and theory: a mixed model of satisfaction, in W.E. Saris, R. Veenhoven, A.C. Scherpenzel and B. Bunting (eds) *A Comparative Study of Satisfaction with Life in Europe*. Budapest: Eötvös University Press.

Sarvimäki, A. (1999) What do we mean by 'quality of life' in our care for people with dementia? *Journal of Dementia Care*, Jan/Feb: 35–7.

Sarvimäki, A. and Stonbock-Hult, B. (2000) Quality of life in old age described as a sense of well-being, meaning and value, *Journal of Advanced Nursing*, 32: 1025–33.

Scales, J. and Scase, R. (2000) *Fit and Fifty: A Report Prepared for the Economic and Social Research Council*. Essex: Institute for Social and Economic Research, University of Essex and the University of Kent at Canterbury.

Schaie, K.W., Wahl, H.W., Mollenkopf, H. and Oswald, F. (eds) (2003) *Aging Independently: Living Arrangements and Mobility*. New York: Springer Publishing Co.

Scharf, T. and Smith, A. (2003) Older people in urban neighbourhoods: addressing the risk of social exclusion in later life, in C. Phillipson, G. Allan and D. Morgan (eds) *Social Networks and Social Exclusion*. Aldershot: Ashgate.

Scheier, M.F. and Carver, C.S. (1985) Optimism, coping and health: assessment and implications of generalised outcome expectancies, *Health Psychology*, 4: 219–47.

Scheier, M.F., Matthews, K.A., Owens, J. *et al.* (1989) Dispositional optimism and recovery from coronary artery bypass surgery: the beneficial effects on physical and psychological well-being, *Journal of Personality and Social Psychology*, 57: 1024–40.

Scheier, M.F., Carver, C.S. and Bridges, M.W. (1994) Distinguishing optimism from neuroticism (and trait anxiety, self-mastery, and self-esteem): a reevaluation of the Life Orientation Test, *Journal of Personality and Social Psychology*, 67: 1063–78.

Schieman, S. (1999) Age and anger, *Journal of Health and Social Behavior*, 40: 273–89.

Schieman, S. and Meersman, S.C. (2004) Neighbourhood problems and health among older adults: received and donated social support and the sense of mastery as effect modifiers, *Journal of Gerontology, Psychological Sciences and Social Sciences*, 59: S89–97.

Schieman, S. and Van Gundy, K. (2000) The personal and social links between age and self-reported empathy, *Social Psychology Quarterly*, 63: 152–74.

Schieman., S., Van Gundy, K. and Taylor, J. (2002) The relationship between age and depressive symptoms: a test of competing explanatory and suppression influences, *Journal of Aging and Health*, 14: 260–85.

Schmitz-Scherzer, R. and Thomae, H. (1983) Constancy and change of behaviour in old age: findings from the Bonn Longitudinal Study of Aging, in K.W. Scraire (ed.) *Longitudinal Studies of Adult Psychological Development*. London: Guilford Press.

Schoenfeld, D.E., Malmrose, L.C., Blazer, D.G. *et al.* (1994) Self-rated health and mortality in the high-functioning elderly – a closer look at healthy individuals: MacArthur field study of successful ageing, *Journal of Gerontology*, 49: M109–15.

Schofield, H. and Bloch, S. (1998) Disability and chronic illness: the role of the family carer, *Medical Journal of Australia*, 169: 405–6.

Schroll, M. (1994) The main pathway in musculoskeletal disability, *Scandinavian Journal of Medicine and Science in Sports*, 4: 3–12.

Schwartz, A.N. (1975) An observation on self-esteem as the linchpin of quality of life for the aged, *The Gerontologist*, 15: 470–2.

Schwartz, N. and Strack, F. (1999) Reports of subjective wellbeing: judgmental processes and their methodological implications, in D. Kanahan, E. Diener and N. Schwartz (eds) *Wellbeing, the foundations of hedonistic psychology*. New York: Russell Sage Foundation.

Schwarzer, R. (1993) *Measurement of Perceived Self-efficacy: Psychometric Scales for Cross-cultural Research*. Berlin: Free University of Berlin, Institute for Psychology.

Sciafa, C.T. and Games, P.A. (1987) Problems with step-wise regression in research on aging and recommended alternatives, *Journal of Gerontology*, 42: 579–83.

Scollon, C.N. and King, L.A. (2004) Is the good life the easy life? *Social Indicators Research*, 68: 127–62.

Seeman, T.E. (2000) Health promoting effects of friends and family on health outcomes in older adults, *American Journal of Health Promotion*, 14: 362–70.

Seeman, T.E., Charpentier, P.A., Berkman, L.F. *et al.* (1994) Predicting changes in physical performance in a high functioning elderly cohort: MacArthur studies of successful aging, *Journal of Gerontology*, 49: M97–108.

Seeman, T.E., Bruce, M.L. and McAvay, G.J. (1996a) Social network characteristics and onset of ADL disability: MacArthur studies of successful aging, *Journal of Gerontology*, 51: S191–200.

Seeman, T.E., McAvay, G. and Merrill, S. *et al.* (1996b) Self-efficacy beliefs and change in cognitive performance: MacArthur studies of successful aging, *Psychology Aging*, 11: 538–51.

Seeman, T.E., Unger, J.B., McAvay, G. and Medes de Leon, C.F. (1999) Self-efficacy beliefs and perceived declines in functional ability: MacArthur studies of successful ageing, *Journal of Gerontology*, 54: 214–22.

Seeman, T.E., Lusignolo, T.M., Albert, M. and Berkman, L. (2001) Social relationships, social support, and patterns of cognitive aging in healthy, high functioning older adults: MacArthur studies of successful ageing, *Health Psychology*, 20: 243–55.

Segerstrom, S.C., Taylor, S.E., Kemeny, M.E. and Fahey, J.L. (1998) Optimism is associated with mood, coping and immune change in response to stress, *Journal of Personality and Social Psychology*, 74: 1546–655.

Seligman, M. (2004) *Authentic Happiness: Using the New Potential for Lasting Fulfilment*. New York: Free Press.

Sen, A.K. (1985) *Commodities and Capabilities*. Amsterdam: North Holland.

Sen, A. (1992) *Inequality Reexamined*. Oxford: Oxford University Press.

Seshamani, M. and Gray, A. (2002) The impact of ageing on expenditures in the National Health Service, *Age and Ageing*, 31: 287–94.

Shanas, E., Townsend, P., Wedderburn, D. *et al.* (1968) *Old People in Three Industrial Societies*. London: Routledge & Kegan Paul.

Sheier, M.F. and Carver, C.S. (1985) Optimism, coping and health: assessment and implications of generalised outcome expectancies, *Health Psychology*, 4: 219–47.

Sheldon, J.H. (1948) *The Social Medicine of Old Age*. Oxford: Oxford University Press.

Sherbourne, C.D. and Stewart, A.L. (1991) The MOS social support survey, *Social Science and Medicine*, 32: 705–14.

Sherif, M.A. (1936) *The Psychology of Social Norms*. New York: Harper.

Sherman, E. and Schiffman, L.G. (1991) Quality of Life (QoL) assessment of older consumers: a retrospective review, *Journal of Business and Psychology*, 6: 107–19.

Siegel, M., Bradley, E.H. and Kasl, S.V. (2003) Self-rated life expectancy as a predictor of mortality: evidence from the HRS and AHEAD surveys, *Gerontology*, 49: 265–71.

Silverstein, M. and Parker, M.G. (2002) Leisure activities and quality of life among the oldest old in Sweden, *Research on Aging*, 25: 528–47.

Singer, E., Garfinkel, R., Cohen, S.M. *et al.* (1976) Mortality and mental health: evidence from the midtown Manhattan re-study, *Social Science and Medicine*, 10: 517–21.

Sirgy, M.J. (1998) Materialism and quality of life, *Social Indicators Research*, 43: 227–60.

Sirgy, M.J. (2002) *The Psychology of Quality of Life*. Dordrecht: Kluwer Academic Publishers.

Sixsmith, A. and Sixsmith, J. (2001) Smart home technologies: meeting whose needs? *Journal of Telemedicine and Telecare*, 6: 190–2.

Skevington, S.M. (1999) Measuring quality of life in Britain: introducing the WHO-QOL-100, *Journal of Psychosocial Research*, 47: 449–59.

Skevington, S.M., Bradshaw, J. and Saxena, S. (1999) Selecting national items for the WHOQOL: conceptual and psychometric considerations, *Social Science and Medicine*, 48: 473–87.

Smith, A.E. (2000) Quality of life: a review, *Education and Ageing*, 15: 419–35.

Spiro, A. and Bossé, R. (2000) Relations between health-related quality of life and well-being: the gerontologist's new clothes, *International Journal of Aging and Human Development*, 50: 297–318.

Sprangers, M.A.G. and Schwartz, C.E. (1999) Integrating response shift into health-related quality of life research: a theoretical model, *Social Science and Medicine*, 48: 150–15.

Staats, S., Heaphey, K., Miller, D., Partlo, C. and Romine, K. (1993) Subjective age and health perceptions of older persons: maintaining the youthful bias in sickness and in health, *International Journal of Aging and Human Development*, 37: 191–203.

Stansfeld, S. (1999) Socal support and social cohesion, in M. Marmot and R.G. Wilkinson (eds) *Social Determinants of Health*. Oxford: Oxford University Press.

Stansfeld, S.A., Fuhrer, R., Shipley, M.J. *et al.* (2002) Psychological distress as a risk factor for coronary heart disease in the Whitehall II study, *International Journal of Epidemiology*, 31: 248–55.

Stastny, P. and Amering, M. (1997) Integrating consumer perspectives in quality of life in research and service planning, in H. Katschnig, H. Freeman and N. Sartorius (eds) *Quality of Life in Mental Disorders*. Chichester: Wiley.

Steitz, J.A. and McClary, A.M. (1988) Subjective age, age identity and middle-age adults, *Experimental Aging Research*, 14: 83–7.

Stenner, P.H.D., Cooper, D. and Skevington, S.M. (2003) Putting the Q into quality of life; the identification of subjective constructions of health-related quality of life using Q methodology, *Social Science and Medicine*, 57: 2161–72.

Stewart, A.L., Sherbourne, C.D. and Brod, M. (1996) Measuring health-related quality of life in older and demented populations, in B. Spilker (ed.) *Quality of Life and Pharmacoeconomics in Clinical Trials*, 2nd edn. Philadelphia, PA: Lippincott-Raven.

Stones, M.L. and Kozma, A. (1980) Issues relating to the usage of conceptualisations of mental constructs employed by gerontologists, *International Journal of Aging and Human Development*, 11: 269–81.

Strawbridge, W.J., Cohen, R.D., Shema, S.J. *et al.* (1996) Successful aging: predictors and associated activities, *American Journal of Epidemiology*, 144: 135–41.

Suchman, E.A. and Phillips, B.S. (1958) An analysis of the validity of health questionnaires, *Social Forces*, 36: 223–32.

Sutton, S. (1998) How ordinary people in Great Britain perceive the health risks of smoking, *Journal of Epidemiology and Community Health*, 52: 338–9.

Suzman, R.M., Willis, D.P. and Manton, K.G. (1992) *The Oldest Old*. New York: Oxford University Press.

Tabachnick, B.G. and Fidell, L.S. (2001) *Using Multivariate Statistics*, 4th edn. Boston: Allyn and Bacon.

Takano, T. and Nakamura, K. (2001) An analysis of health levels and various indicators of urban environments for Healthy Cities projects, *Journal of Epidemiology and Community Health*, 55: 263–70.

Tate, R.B., Leedine, L. and Cuddy, T.E. (2003) Definition of successful aging by elderly Canadian males: the Manitoba follow-up study, *The Gerontologist*, 43: 735–44.

Taylor, R. and Ford, G. (1983) Inequality in old age: an examination of age, sex and class differences in a sample of community elderly, *Ageing and Society*, 3: 183–208.

Taylor, S.E. (1983) Adjustment to threatening events: a theory of cognitive adaptation, *American Psychologist*, 38: 1161–73.

Taylor, S.E., Wood, J.V. and Lichtman, R.R. (1983) It could be worse: selective evaluation as a response to victimisation, *Journal of Social Issues*, 39: 19–40.

Tester, S., Downs, M. and Hubbard, G. (2000) Research in progress: exploring perceptions of quality of life of frail older people, *Generations Review, Journal of the British Society of Gerontology*, 10: 17–18.

Thane, P. (2000) *Old Age in English History: Past Experiences, Present Issues*. Oxford: Oxford University Press.

Thoits, P.A. (1982) Conceptual, methodological and theoretical problems in studying social support as a buffer against life stress, *Journal of Health and Social Behavior*, 23: 145–59.

Thomas, W.C. (1981) The expectation gap and the stereotype of the stereotype: images of old people, *Gerontologist*, 21: 402–7.

Tobin, S.S. and Lieberman, M.A. (1976) *Last Home for the Aged*. San Francisco: Jossey-Bass.

Tornstam, L. (1997) Gerotranscendence in a broad cross-sectional perspective, *Journal of Aging and Identity*, 2: 17–36.

Torres, S. (1999) A culturally-relevant theoretical framework for the study of successful ageing, *Ageing and Society*, 19: 33–51.

Torres, S. (2003) A preliminary empirical test of a culturally relevant theoretical framework for the study of successful aging, *Journal of Cross-Cultural Gerontology*, 18: 79–100.

Townsend, P. (1957) *The Family Life of Old People*. London: Routledge & Kegan Paul.

Townsend, P. (1979) *Poverty in the United Kingdom*. Harmondsworth: Pelican.

Townsend, P. and Davidson, N. (1982) *Inequalities in Health, The Black Report*. Harmondsworth: Pelican.

Troen, B.R. (2003) The biology of ageing, *Mount Sinai Journal of Medicine*, 70: 3–22.

Tunstall, J. (1966) *Old and Alone*. London: Routledge & Kegan Paul.

United Nations (1994) *Information on Social Development Publications and Indicators in the United Nations System*, working paper no. 7. New York: United Nations.

Usui, W.M., Thomas, J.K. and Durig, K.R. (1985) Socioeconomic comparisons and life satisfaction of elderly adults, *Journal of Gerontology*, 40: 110–14.

Vaillant, G.E. (1990) Avoiding negative life outcomes: evidence from a forty five year study, in P.B. Baltes and M.M. Baltes (eds) *Successful Ageing: Perspectives from the Behavioral Sciences*. New York: Cambridge University Press.

Vaillant, G.E. (2002) *Aging Well: Surprising Guideposts to a Happier Life from the Landmark Harvard Study of Adult Development*. Boston, MA: Little, Brown.

Veenhoven, R. (1991) Is happiness relative? *Social Indicators Research*, 24: 1–34.

Veenhoven, R. (1993) *Happiness in Nations: Subjective Appreciation of Life in 56 Nations 1946–1992*. Rotterdam: RISBO, Erasmus University of Rotterdam.

Veenhoven, R. (1994) Is happiness a trait? Tests of the theory that a better society does not make us any happier, *Social Indicators Research*, 32: 101–62.

Veenhoven, R. (1996) The study of life-satisfaction, in W.E. Saris, R. Veenhoven, A.C. Scherpenzeel and B. Bunting (eds) *A Comparative Study of Satisfaction with Life in Europe*. Budapest: Eötvös University Press.

Veenhoven, R. (1997) Progrés dans la compréhension du bonheur, *Revue Québécoise de Psychologie*, 18: 29–74.

Veenhoven, R. (1999) Quality of life in individualistic society, *Social Indicators Research*, 48: 157–86.

Veenhoven, R. (2000) The four qualities of life: ordering concepts and measures of the good life, *Journal of Happiness Studies*, 1: 1–39.

Veenhoven, R. (2002) Why social policy needs subjective indicators, *Social Indicators Research*, 58: 33–45.

Verbrugge, L. (1985) An epidemiological profile of older women, in M. Haug, A. Ford and M. Sheafor (eds) *The Physical and Mental Health of Aged Women*. New York: Springer.

Verbrugge, L. (1989) The twain meet: empirical explanations of sex differences in health and mortality, *Journal of Health and Social Behavior*, 30: 282–304.

Victor, C., Scambler, S., Bond, J. and Bowling, A. (2000) Being alone in later life: loneliness, social isolation and living alone, *Reviews in Clinical Gerontology*, 10: 407–17.

Victor, C.V., Scambler, S.J., Bond, J. and Bowling, A. (2004) Loneliness in later life, in A. Walker and C. Hagen Hennessy (eds) *Growing Older: Quality of Life in Older Age*. Maidenhead: Open University Press.

von Faber, M., Bootsma-van der Weil, A., van Exel, E. *et al.* (2001) Successful aging in the oldest old: who can be characterised as successfully aged? *Archives of Internal Medicine*, 161: 2694–700.

Wahl, H.W. (2001) Environmental influences on aging and behavior, in J.E. Birren and K.W. Schaie (eds) *Handbook of the Psychology of Aging*, 5th edn. San Diego, CA: Academic Press.

Wahl, H.W. and Mollenkopf, H. (2003) Impact of everyday technology in the home environment on older adult's quality of life, in K.W. Schaie and N. Charness (eds) *Impact of Technology on Successful Ageing*. New York: Springer.

Wahl, H.W. and Weisman, G.D. (2003) Environmental gerontology at the beginning of the new millennium: reflections on its historical, empirical, and theoretical development, *The Gerontologist*, 43: 616–27.

Wahl, H.W., Scheidt, R. and Windley, P. (eds) (2003) *Annual Review of Gerontology and Geriatrics: Ageing in Context – Socio-physical Environments*, vol. 23. New York: Springer.

Walker, A. (1981) Towards a political economy of old age, *Ageing and Society*, 1: 73–94.

Walker, A. (1993) Poverty and inequality in old age, in J. Bond, P. Coleman and S. Peace (eds) *Ageing in Society: An Introduction to Social Gerontology*, 2nd edn. London: Sage.

Walker, A. (2002) *Extending Quality of Life in Old Age (EQUAL)*. Sheffield: Department of Social Policy, University of Sheffield.

Walker, A. (2005) Quality of life in old age in Europe, in A. Walker (ed.) *Growing Older in Europe*. Maidenhead: Open University Press.

Walker, A. (in press) Re-examining the political economy of aging: understanding the structure/agency tension, in J. Baars, D. Dannefer and A. Walker (eds) *Aging, Globalization and Inequality*. New York: Baywood.

Walker, A. and Maltby, T. (1997) *Ageing Europe*. Buckingham: Open University Press.

Walker, A. and Walker, C. (2005) The UK: quality of life in old age, in A. Walker (ed.) *Growing Older in Europe*. Maidenhead: Open University Press.

Walker, A., Maher, J., Coulthard, M. *et al.* (2001) *Living in Britain: Results from the 2000 General Household Survey*. London: The Stationery Office.

Walker, K., Macbride, A. and Vachon, M.L.S. (1997) Social support networks and the crisis of bereavement, *Social Science and Medicine*, 11: 34–41.

Wang, H.X., Karp, A., Winblad, B. and Fratiglioli, L. (2002) Late-life engagement in social and leisure activities is associated with a decreased risk of dementia: a longitudinal study from the Kungsholmen Project, *American Journal of Epidemiology*, 155: 1081–7.

Wanless, D. (2002) *Securing our Future Health: Taking a Long Term View – Final Report*. London: HM Treasury.

Ware, J.E. and Bayliss, M.S. (2003) The future of item 'banking': who should make deposits and how should they be used, *Quality of Life Newsletter*, Fall: 15–18.

Ware, J.E. and Sherbourne, C.D. (1992) The MOS 36-item short-form health survey (SF-36): I – Conceptual framework and item selection, *Medical Care*, 30: 473–83.

Ware, J.E, Snow, K.K., Kosinski, M. and Gandek, B. (1993) *SF-36 Health Survey*. Boston, MA: New England Medical Centre.

Warr, P.B. (1999) Well-being and the workplace, in D. Kahnerman, E. Diener and N. Schwarz (eds) *Well-being: The Foundations of Hedonic Psychology*. New York: Sage.

Waters, W.E., Heikinen, E. and Dontas, A.S. (1998) *Health, Lifestyles and Services for the Elderly*. Copenhagen: World Health Organization.

Watkins, F., Bendel, N., Scott-Samual, A. and Whitehead, M. (2002) Through a glass darkly: what should public health observatories be observing? *Journal of Public Health Medicine*, 24: 160–4.

Webster, N., Gow, J., Gilhooly, M. *et al.* (2002) Transport barriers to activity in old age, in T. Maltby, R. Littlechild, J. La Fontaine, S. Hunter and P. Brannelly (eds) *Active Ageing: Myth or Reality?* Proceedings of the British Society of Gerontology, 31st Annual Conference. Paisley: Centre for Gerontology and Health Studies: University of Paisley.

Weidekamp-Maicher, M. (2001) *Quality of Life in Old Age: German Impulses*. Dortmund: University of Dortmund.

Weinstein, N.D. (1980) Unrealistic optimism about future events, *Journal of Personality and Social Psychology*, 34: 806–20.

Wenger, G.C. (1984a) *The Supportive Network: Coping with Old Age*. London: Allen & Unwin.

Wenger, G.C. (1984b) Adapting to old age in rural Britain, *International Journal of Aging and Human Development*, 19: 289–301.

Wenger, G.C. (1989) Support networks in old age: constructing a typology, in M. Jeffreys (ed.) *Growing Old in the Twentieth Century*. London: Routledge.

Wenger, G.C. (1992) Morale in old age: a review of the evidence, *International Journal of Geriatric Psychiatry*, 7: 699–708.

Wenger, G.C. (1996) Social networks and gerontology, *Reviews in Clinical Gerontology*, 6: 285–93.

Wenger, G.C. and Shahtahmasebi, S. (1990) Variations in support networks: implications for social policy, in M.J. Mogey, P. Somlai and J. Trost (eds) *Aiding and Aging: The Coming Crisis*. Westport, CT: Greenwood Press.

Wenger, G.C., Scott, A. and Patterson, N. (2000) How important is parenthood? Childlessness and support in old age in England, *Ageing and Society*, 20: 161–82.

Wentowski, G. (1981) Reciprocity and the coping strategies of older people: cultural dimensions of network building, *Gerontologist*, 21: 600–9.

Wetle, T. (1991) Autonomy as a factor in quality of life in the frail elderly: resident decision making, in J.E. Birren, J.E. Lubben, J.C. Rowe and D.E. Deutchman (eds) *The Concept and Measurement of Quality of Life in the Frail Elderly*. San Diego, CA: Academic Press.

Wheeler, L. and Miyake, K. (1992) Social comparison in everyday life, *Journal of Personality and Social Psychology*, 62: 760–73.

Whitehead, M. (1987) *The Health Divide: Inequalities in Health in the 1980s*. London: Health Education Council.

WHOQOL Group (1993) *Measuring Quality of Life: The Development of the World Health Organisation Quality of Life Instrument (WHOQOL)*. Geneva: WHO.

Wilkinson, R. (1996) *Unhealthy Societies – The Afflictions of Inequality*. London: Routledge.

Willcox, B.J., Willcox, C. and Suzuki, M. (2001) *The Okinawa Program: How the World's Longest-lived People Achieve Everlasting Health – and How You Can Too*. New York: Clarkson Potter.

Wilson, S.R. and Benner, L.A. (1971) The effects of self-esteem and situation upon comparison choices during ability evaluation, *Sociometry*, 34: 381–97.

Wingo, L. and Evans, A. (1978) *Public Economics and the Quality of Life*. Baltimore, MD: Johns Hopkins University Press.

Wood, C. (1987) Are happy people healthier? Discussion paper, *Journal of the Royal Society of Medicine*, 80: 354–6.

Wood, J.V., Taylor, S.E. and Lichtman, R.R. (1985) Social comparison in adjustment to breast cancer, *Journal of Personality and Social Psychology*, 49: 1169–83.

Wood, V., Wylie, M.L. and Scheafor, B. (1969) An analysis of a short self-report measure of life satisfaction: correlation with rater judgements, *Journal of Gerontology*, 24: 465–9.

World Health Organization (1948) *Preamble to the Constitution of the World Health Organization as Adopted by the International Health Conference, New York 19–22 June 1946.* Geneva: WHO.

World Health Organization (1980) *International Classification of Impairments, Disabilities and Handicaps.* Geneva: WHO.

World Health Organization (1998) *ICIDH-2 – International Classification of Impairments, Activities and Participation: A Manual of Dimensions of Disablement and Functioning.* Geneva: WHO.

World Health Organization (2001) *International Classification of Functioning, Disability and Health.* Geneva: WHO.

World Health Organization (2002) *Active Ageing: A Policy Framework.* Geneva: WHO.

Wright, F. (2004) *Older and Colder – The Views of Older People Experiencing Difficulties Keeping Warm in Winter.* London: British Gas Help the Aged Partnership.

Yngwe, A., Diderichsen, F., Whitehead, M. *et al.* (2001) The role of income differences in explaining social inequalities in self-rated health in Sweden and Britain, *Journal of Epidemiology and Community Health,* 55: 556–61.

Young, M. and Wilmott, P. (1957) *Family and Kinship in East London.* London: Routledge & Kegan Paul.

Zautra, A. and Hempel, A. (1984) Subjective well-being and physical health: a narrative literature review with suggestions for future research, *International Journal of Aging and Human Development,* 19: 95–110.

Ziller, R.C. (1974) Self-other orientation and quality of life, *Social Indicators Research,* 1: 301–27.

Zizzi, A., Barry, M.M. and Cochrane, R. (1998) A mediational model of quality of life for individuals with severe mental health problems, *Psychological Medicine,* 28: 1221–30.

Index

Note on using this index: the methods of the study are indexed in alphabetical order under *Quality of life survey methods* and the results are indexed alphabetically under *Quality of life survey results*. Theories of quality of life are indexed under *Quality of life models and measures*. The start of each index list is marked in **bold**.

Related books from Open University Press

Purchase from www.openup.co.uk or order through your local bookseller

UNDERSTANDING QUALITY OF LIFE IN OLD AGE

Alan Walker (ed)

This book considers key findings from the Economic and Social Research Council (ESRC) funded Growing Older Programme (1999-2004) and presents these in a lively thematic format. It discusses topics such as environment, family, bereavement, identity, and social interaction and describes key concepts and measures. Using data drawn from a range of different research projects, the chapters illustrate considerable methodological diversity to capture a broad picture of quality of life for older people. Key implications for future research on quality of life in older age are also proposed.

The book is a companion volume to *Growing Older: Quality of Life in Old Age* edited by Alan Walker and Catherine Hagan Hennessy and is recommended reading on a range of advanced undergraduate and postgraduate courses including social gerontology, social work, sociology and social policy.

Contributors:
Sara Arber, John Baldock, Kate M. Bennett, David Blane, Ann Bowling, Elizabeth Breeze, Jabeer Butt, Lynda Clarke, Peter Coleman, Kate Davidson, Murna Downs, Maria Evandrou, Ken Gilhooly, Mary Gilhooly, Jane Gow, Jan Hadlow, Catherine Hagan Hennessy, Paul Higgs, Caroline Holland, Georgina M. Hughes, Martin Hyde, Leonie Kellaher, Mary Maynard, Kevin McKee, F. McKiernan, Christopher McKevitt, Marie Mills, Jo Moriarty, James Nazroo, Sheila Peace, Thomas Scharf, Philip T. Smith, Peter Speck, Susan Tester, Christina Victor, Alan Walker, Peter Warr, Lorna Warren, Dick Wiggins, Fiona Wilson.

Contents:
Investigating quality of life in the Growing Older Programme - Quality of life: meaning and measurement - Dimensions of the inequalities in quality of life in older age - Getting out and about - Family and economic roles - Social involvement: aspects of gender and ethnicity - Social isolation and loneliness - Frailty, identity and the quality of later life - Identity, meaning and social support - Elderly bereaved spouses: issues of belief, well-being and support - Conclusion: from research to action - Index.

c.192pp   0 335 21523 8 (Paperback)   0 335 21524 6 (Hardback)

GROWING OLDER IN EUROPE

Alan Walker (ed)

Growing Older in Europe is a companion volume to the other books in the Growing Older series and provides the first comparative European perspective on ageing. The comparisons demonstrate that although similar quality of later life issues are faced by older people in different European Union countries, the policy and service contexts are significantly different, as are the research traditions.

Based on systematic reviews of evidence from the United Kingdom, Germany, Italy, the Netherlands and Sweden, the book provides a unique resource for anyone interested in the rapidly growing field of ageing.

Written by prominent experts, the research evidence highlights topics such as:

- physical and mental health
- the environments of ageing
- employment and income
- family and support networks
- participation and social integration
- good practice in the promotion of quality of life

The book is key reading for specialists, including students, practitioners and policy makers, as well as lay people with an interest in the fields of social gerontology, sociology and social policy.

Contributors:
Lars Andersson, Beitske Bouwman, Kees Knipscheer, Giovanni Lamura, Annemarie Peters, Francesca Polverini, Monika Reichert, Carol Walker, Manuela Weidekamp-Maicher.

Contents:
Contributors – Preface – Quality of life in old age in Europe – Part I. Quality of life in old age: definitions, environments and socio-economic aspects – Germany: quality of life in old age I – Italy: quality of life in old age I – The Netherlands: quality of life in old age I – Sweden: quality of life in old age I – The UK: quality of life in old age I – Part II. Quality of life in old age: participation, social support and subjective wellbeing – Germany: quality of life in old age II – Italy: quality of life in old age II – The Netherlands: quality of life in old age II – Sweden: quality of life in old age II – The UK: quality of life in old age II – References – Index

312pp   0 335 21513 0 (Paperback)   0 335 21514 9 (Hardback)

QUALITY OF LIFE AND OLDER PEOPLE

John Bond and Lynne Corner

Quality of Life and Older People provides a critical approach to the conceptualization and measurement of quality of life in social gerontology and health and social care research. The book re-examines what we mean by 'quality of life' in a post-modern world, and examines the impact of continuous personal and social changes on the lives of older people.

The authors explore ideas about quality of life in social gerontological literature, and attempt to describe the experiences of older people through both their own self description and analysts representations of their experiences. They present a critique of existing social science theories underpinning conceptions of quality of life, and address operational issues for the use of quality of life in social gerontological research.

This book forms part of the *Rethinking Ageing Series*, and is suitable for undergraduate and post-graduate students of social gerontology, social policy, education, health, medicine and social work, as well as policy makers and practitioners working with older people; researchers and professionals.

Contents:
Series editor's preface – Copyright acknowledgements – Preface and acknowledgements – What is quality of life? – Talking about quality of life – Environment and quality of life – Quality of life and the post-modern world – Explaining quality of life – Assessing quality of life – Rethinking quality of life – References – Index.

160pp   0 335 20872 X (Paperback)   0 335 20873 8 (Hardback)

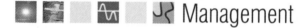
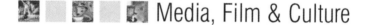
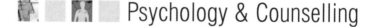
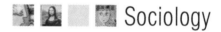
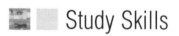
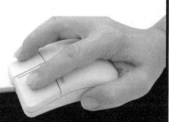
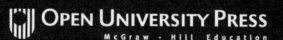